MCQs for MRCP Part 1

For Churchill Livingstone

Commissioning Editor Laurence Hunter
Copy Editors Paul Singleton, Susan Beasley
Project Controller Nancy Arnott
Sales Promotion Executive Duncan Jones

MCQs for MRCP Part 1—General Medicine

Michael J. Ford
MBChB (Hons) MD FRCP (Edin)
Consultant Physician
Eastern General Hospital, Edinburgh, UK

David M. Matthews
MBChB FRCP (Edin) FRCP (Glasg)
Consultant Physician
Stonehouse and Hairmyres Hospitals, Lanarkshire, UK

Second Edition

CHURCHILL LIVINGSTONE
EDINBURGH HONG KONG LONDON MADRID MELBOURNE NEW YORK AND TOKYO 1995

CHURCHILL LIVINGSTONE
Medical Division of Longman Group Limited

Distributed in the United States of America by Churchill
Livingstone Inc., 650 Avenue of the Americas, New York, N.Y.
10011, and by associated companies, branches and
representatives throughout the world.

First edition 1986
Second edition 1995

ISBN 0 443 05083 X

British Library Cataloguing in Publication Data
A catalogue record for this book is available from the British Library.

Library of Congress Cataloging in Publication Data
A catalog record for this book is available from the Library of Congress.

First edition compiled and edited by
Michael J. Ford and E. Fiona Nicol
and published under the title
MCQs for MRCP Part 1.

The
publisher's
policy is to use
**paper manufactured
from sustainable forests**

Produced by Longman Singapore Publishers (Pte) Ltd.
Printed in Singapore.

Contents

Preface

The MRCP Part 1 examination is the first substantial hurdle of the aspiring physician in the United Kingdom and many young doctors approach this with considerable apprehension. We have addressed this problem in the contents of this book which aims to direct candidates in the correct run-up to the examination.

The book is organized in chapters with appropriate numbers of questions corresponding to those asked in the General Medical examination, taking into account the removal of specific paediatric questions into a separate test from October 1993. Many new questions in clinical science and practice have been introduced.

We wish to thank Mrs Mary Craw for her valued secretarial assistance in preparing the manuscript.

Lanark, 1995   D. M. M.
Edinburgh, 1995   M. F.

Introduction

The MRCP (Part 1) examination is the first part of an entrance examination for higher medical training in the United Kingdom. The examination is easy to fail without a broad and detailed knowledge of clinical medicine and the related basic sciences. A total of four attempts are allowed, and a bad fail will delay the next attempt for 1 year.

Candidates are required to answer 300 multiple-choice questions in 150 minutes. Each MCQ is of the true/false/don't know variety. There are 60 stems or statements with five items in relation to each stem. The items may be unrelated to one another, but all are related to the stem. For example:

In diabetes mellitus
A the blood sugar is elevated
B children are not affected
C hypertriglyceridaemia is usually resistant to insulin therapy
D fructosuria is a characteristic finding
E stiff joints are a recognized long-term complication

(Correct answers are: A and E.)

Diabetes mellitus is a common condition, and all physicians should know that the blood sugar is elevated and that children are certainly affected. Items C and D make candidates think about the biochemical defects, and require a sound grasp of basic biochemistry. Candidates with a specialist knowledge of diabetes will know that arthropathy is a rare, but characteristic, feature of patients with long-standing insulin-dependent diabetes mellitus.

In the typical examination of 60 stem questions, you can expect to see five questions on clinical pharmacology and four questions each on the nine major medical specialities (i.e. cardiology, respiratory medicine, gastroenterology, endocrinology, neurology, rheumatology, nephrology, haematology, and infectious diseases). There will be ten questions covering the minor medical specialities, including dermatology, oncology, psychiatry, geriatric medicine, genito-urinary medicine, clinical and molecular genetics, and occupational medicine. The remaining nine questions comprise principally basic science questions in immunology, molecular medicine, statistics, epidemiology, clinical anatomy, physiology, biochemistry, microbiology and pathology. Basic science items are usually closely integrated with more clinically-related questions. It should be remembered, however, that this formula is a crude estimate of the relative contributions from each area of medicine. Nonetheless, it should give candidates a sufficient idea as to how best to prepare themselves for the examination.

Candidates should be ready to answer questions in clinical pharmacology concerning toxicology, drug interactions, drug-induced disease, the use of drugs in patients with concomitant hepatic or renal disease, and the use of drugs during pregnancy or the post-partum period. Basic pharmacological concepts associated with pharmacodynamics and pharmacokinetics are likely to be assessed in the examination. Amongst the questions relating to the major specialities, the guiding theme will be that of clinical relevance such that there will be many questions concerning the clinical and investigational findings in specific disease and the related items of basic science necessary for an understanding of the disorder.

Preparation
In preparing for the examination, there is no substitute for detailed study of all areas of clinical medicine. For many, this cannot be achieved without at least 3 months of regular reading sessions. Some find it useful to meet in groups and prepare topics for discussion, including MCQs, beforehand. In this way, areas of difficulty in understanding can often be resolved. In addition, prospective candidates will feel more confident that they are ready to take the examination. If, however, after enrolling for the examination, a candidate does not feel adequately prepared, he/she would be better advised to withdraw from the examination, saving time and money, rather than proceeding in a speculative way on the off chance of passing the examination.

Reading a standard textbook of medicine is important in preparation for the examination, and in this regard, the textbooks of medicine by Souhami and Moxham, Kumar and Clarke, and *Davidson's Principles and Practice* are appropriate. Larger textbooks, such as Harrison's *Principles of Internal Medicine* or *Oxford Textbook of Medicine,* are useful to clarify reference items, but too large and comprehensive to be appropriate day-to-day manuals. *The British National Formulary*, published twice yearly, is well worth reading, particularly the text at the beginning of each section. In addition, books of MCQs can be particularly helpful in identifying areas of knowledge requiring more work. In tackling multiple-choice questions, there are certain helpful ground rules, and these include:

READ THE QUESTION VERY CAREFULLY
We all misread words occasionally, but particularly when under stress. It is easy to see how chlorpropamide and chlorpromazine can be confused in the context of an examination.
ASK YOURSELF WHY THE QUESTION IS BEING POSED IN THIS WAY
This can be a useful way of approaching questions, because what appears to be an obvious question with an obvious answer may be less obvious on careful re-reading. The wording of the question has been designed to help you avoid an erroneous interpretation of the

question, not to trick you. For instance, the answer to the question 'Which of the following features favour a diagnosis of myocardial infarction rather than acute pulmonary embolism?' is very different from the answer to the question 'Which of the following features favour a diagnosis of acute pulmonary embolism rather than myocardial infarction?'.

LOGICAL REASONING IS BETTER THAN BLIND GUESSWORK
Even the best informed do not know all the answers. It is very important that candidates do not guess because of the negative marking system which penalizes mistakes. Nonetheless, it is often possible to deduce an answer by reasoned and careful logic, even when one cannot recall reading the answer to such a question in any text.

DON'T BE FRIGHTENED TO ADMIT THAT YOU DON'T KNOW
It is often difficult to admit ignorance and, under pressure, the temptation is simply to guess. If the question concerns an area of knowledge with which you are totally unfamiliar and there is no reasonable way in which you may logically deduce an answer, DON'T GUESS, but record your answer 'Don't know'.

The wording in some multiple-choice questions may appear difficult to those who have no experience of MCQs. The words 'always', 'never', or 'invariably' are rarely seen in an MCQ examination, as they beg the answer 'false', since the practice of medicine does not often deal with such a degree of certainty. Similarly, the words 'can' or 'may' are unusual in MCQs given that most things are possible in medicine. When such words are seen, therefore, the correct answer to the question is more often false than true.

The word 'pathognomonic' means that the occurrence of a sign or symptom is 100% specific to the disease stated and never occurs in the absence of the disease. If the words 'frequently', 'commonly' or 'usually' are used, this means that the symptoms or signs stated are a feature in at least 50% of instances. When the words 'characteristically' or 'typically' are used, this means that such symptoms or signs may not occur in the majority of instances, but when they do occur, they are of considerable diagnostic or therapeutic significance. Finally, the word 'recognized' means that the occurrence of a sign or symptom has been reported in the medical literature, though it may be a rare event.

The marking system
Candidates are awarded one mark for a correct answer, and one mark is deducted for an incorrect answer. No mark is deducted for the answer 'Don't know'. It is, therefore, possible for a candidate to have a negative score. In general, at each sitting of the examination, only 30% will pass. The score required to pass varies with each examination, but is usually of the order of 55%. Clearly, the more questions answered without guessing, the more likely a candidate is to pass the examination. Candidates who answer more than 250 questions are much more likely to have guessed than those who

answer 200 questions. A score of 170+ is very likely to secure a pass, whilst the score of ≤ 160 is very unlikely to achieve a pass. Successful candidates have usually answered no more than 240 of the 300 items. If in so doing, 60 of the 240 items answered involved an element of reasoned guesswork (and at least 50% of the guesses were correct), the minimum score of 180 (240 − 60 = 180; 60%) would be sufficient to secure a pass.

The day of the examination
Make sure that you have had a good night's sleep prior to the examination, and arrive in good time at the examination centre. Remember to append your name and examination number to the answer card. It is surprising the number of candidates who fail to do this appropriately. At the appointed time, carefully read through the entire question booklet methodically, recording your answers (true/false/don't know) beside each item in the margin of the question book. When you have completed the examination, review all items marked 'don't know'. Subsequent questions may have facilitated the recall of the appropriate answer or brought to mind items of knowledge which, by the use of deductive reasoning, will help determine the correct answer to the question which initially posed significant difficulties. Transfer your answers carefully to the answer card using the appropriate soft-leaded pencil. Remember that the answer card is marked by an optical scanner; take care, therefore, not to smudge the shaded boxes when recording your answers on the answer sheet. When you have carefully reviewed all the questions and your answers at least twice and you can attempt no more questions in the 'don't know' section, hand in your answer card and leave the examination. Repeatedly reviewing your answers may be counterproductive and evoke unwarranted anxiety about their correctness. In this regard, your first thoughts are often the most accurate.

Good luck!

How to use this book

The text consists of questions on the left-hand pages and answers with explanations on the right. Readers may wish to cover the right-hand page as they answer the questions.

Clinical pharmacology, therapeutics & toxicology

1 **Abrupt drug withdrawal following prolonged administration can be expected to produce clinically significant reactions in the following therapies**
A clonidine
B corticosteroids
C propranolol
D lorazepam
E warfarin

2 **Interstitial pneumonitis is a recognized consequence of treatment with**
A nitrofurantoin
B aspirin
C methysergide
D bleomycin
E cephaloridine

3 **Drugs which induce bronchospasm include**
A aspirin
B penicillin
C disodium cromoglycate
D indomethacin
E distigmine bromide

1 A **True**   hypertensive crisis and tachycardia
   B **True**   adrenocortical insufficiency and increased disease activity
   C **True**   supersensitivity of beta-adrenergic receptors may result in hypertensive crisis and severe angina or myocardial infarction
   D **True**   confusion, convulsions and conditions resembling delirium tremens
   E **False**   no adverse effects following withdrawal

2 A **True**   usually acute hypersensitivity but some progress to pulmonary fibrosis
   B **False**
   C **True**   more often produces pleural fibrosis and effusions
   D **True**   also produced by busulphan, cyclophosphamide and melphalan
   E **False**

3 A **True**   may produce acute bronchospasm or chronic asthma and is commoner in late-onset asthmatics (non-atopic)
   B **True**   usually occurs in the context of anaphylactic reactions
   C **True**   usually a direct irritant effect but occasionally occurs in the context of anaphylactic reactions
   D **True**   aspirin-sensitive asthmatics are usually also sensitive to many of the non-steroidal anti-inflammatory drugs
   E **True**   parasympathomimetics including edrophonium, neostigmine and pilocarpine may aggravate asthma

4   Aminoglycoside antibiotics
   A   should be monitored by measurement of their plasma
         concentration
   B   all produce ototoxicity
   C   are well absorbed, given orally
   D   penetrate the CSF readily
   E   produce ventilatory failure in sensitive individuals

5   Adverse effects of treatment with ciprofloxacin include
   A   anaphylaxis
   B   crystalluria
   C   discoloration of teeth in children
   D   convulsions
   E   pseudomembranous colitis

6   Factors determining the bioavailability of drugs include
   A   tablet disintegration time
   B   gastrointestinal motility
   C   first-pass hepatic metabolism
   D   drug dosage
   E   intraluminal gastric pH

**7   The following drugs precipitate haemolysis in patients with
     glucose-6-phosphate dehydrogenase deficiency**
   A   aspirin
   B   primaquine
   C   propranolol
   D   dapsone
   E   trimethoprim

4 A **True** essential if high doses or treatment are given for longer than 7 days

B **True** streptomycin and gentamicin predominantly produce vestibular effects, amikacin and vancomycin auditory effects and tobramycin affects both equally. Netilmicin has less ototoxic effects

C **False** less than 1% is absorbed following oral administration, although absorption can occur in liver failure and inflammatory bowel disease

D **False** because of their polar nature, penetration of the CSF and ocular fluids is very limited

E **True** because of neuromuscular blockage, patients under anaesthesia and patients with myasthenia gravis are at special risk

---

5 A **True** especially in patients with AIDS

B **True** adequate fluid intake important

C **False** occurs with tetracycline

D **True** a risk of 4-quinolone antibiotics especially if coexistent use of non-steroidal anti-inflammatory drugs

E **True** occurs following treatment with most broad-spectrum antibiotics and is related to the overgrowth of *Clostridium difficile*

---

6 A **True** the bioavailability of any drug is expressed by the ratio of area under the absorption curve after oral/parenteral administration. Any factor delaying drug absorption or entry into the systemic circulation will therefore adversely affect the bioavailability

B **True**
C **True**
D **False**
E **True**

---

7 A **True** any drug whose metabolism involves a major oxidative pathway is likely to induce haemolysis in individuals with G6PD deficiency

B **True** it is dose-related and, for this reason, acidosis and infection also aggravate the condition

C **False**
D **True**
E **False**

8 Malignant hyperthermia is a recognized complication of treatment with
A aspirin
B suxamethonium
C halothane
D trichlorethylene
E dantrolene

9 Indomethacin therapy
A increases amyloid deposition in rheumatoid arthritis
B is contraindicated in the treatment of osteo-arthrosis
C reduces hepatic blood flow in cirrhosis
D should be avoided in patients with renal disease
E enhances uric acid excretion by the kidneys

10 Oral therapy with activated charcoal is a useful adjunct in the management of poisoning with
A paracetamol
B carbamazepine
C theophylline
D mefenamic acid
E lithium

11 The following drugs reduce the efficacy of oral anticoagulants
A phenobarbitone
B rifampicin
C carbamazepine
D griseofulvin
E ethyl alcohol

12 The clinical features of tricyclic antidepressant overdosage include
A paralytic ileus
B convulsions
C hallucinations
D urinary retention
E supraventricular tachycardia

8 A **False** inherited as an autosomal dominant trait, the condition may be linked with other myotonic disorders. Intracellular transport of calcium is deranged and generalized muscular contraction may be provoked by many anaesthetic agents
   B **True**
   C **True**
   D **True**
   E **False** may be used in the treatment of the condition

9 A **False** indomethacin is a potent non-steroidal anti-inflammatory agent. Its use should be reserved for patients who have failed to respond to other safer drugs. The use of NSAI drugs should be avoided in renal disease because the inhibition of prostaglandin synthesis may seriously impair renal blood flow; similarly, hepatic blood flow may be critically impaired in hepatic cirrhosis
   B **False**
   C **True**
   D **True**
   E **True**

10 A **False** acetylcysteine or methionine is the treatment of choice
    B **True**
    C **True**
    D **False** convulsions occur and are treated with diazepam
    E **False**

11 A **True** ⎫ all these drugs stimulate microsomal enzyme induction and increase the metabolism of oral anticoagulants, reducing their efficacy
    B **True** ⎪
    C **True** ⎬
    D **True** ⎭
    E **False** enhanced anticoagulant effect

12 A **True** tricyclic antidepressants exert anti-cholinergic effects in overdosage, giving rise to all of these effects together with blurred vision, dry mouth, mydriasis and a flushed, hot but dry skin
    B **True**
    C **True**
    D **True**
    E **True**

13   In thyrotoxicosis, propranolol therapy
    A   impairs myocardial contractility
    B   decreases the uptake of iodine by the thyroid gland
    C   reduces the amplitude and frequency of thyrotoxic tremor
    D   is principally excreted unchanged in the urine
    E   reduces sweating

14   Colchicine
    A   inhibits leucocyte migration
    B   is an effective uricosuric drug
    C   is the drug of choice in the prophylaxis of gout
    D   will relieve acute attacks of gout within 12 hours
    E   commonly gives rise to diarrhoea

15   The following drugs are known to precipitate acute intermittent porphyria
    A   chlorpromazine
    B   oestrogens
    C   griseofulvin
    D   barbiturates
    E   pethidine

16   Drugs which inhibit microsomal enzyme function during chronic administration include
    A   phenobarbitone
    B   valproic acid
    C   ethyl alcohol
    D   allopurinol
    E   disulfiram

13 A **True** propranolol may precipitate cardiac failure in patients with thyrotoxic heart disease and digitalization is recommended
   B **False** potassium perchlorate blocks iodine uptake by the thyroid and carbimazole blocks the iodination process of hormonogenesis
   C **True** beta-blockade will reduce the adrenergic stimulation of physiological tremor
   D **False** propranolol is metabolized in the liver
   E **True** sweat gland innervation has both cholinergic and adrenergic receptors

14 A **True** inhibits leucocyte migration, the production of leucotactic factors, and cell division
   B **False** no effect on urate clearance
   C **False** not recommended unless all other measures have been tried. It is of some value in patients in heart failure or taking warfarin
   D **True** usually effective within 12 hours of administration
   E **True** nausea, vomiting, abdominal pain and diarrhoea are common after a latent period of several hours

15 A **False** any drug stimulating microsomal enzyme induction will precipitate severe attacks in acute intermittent porphyria
   B **True** ⎤ drugs known to be safe include penicillin, pethidine, diazepam, diamorphine, acetylsalicylic acid and
   C **True** ⎟ chlorpromazine. The erythropoietic porphyrias are not aggravated by drug therapy (with the exception of drugs which induce photosensitivity)
   D **True** ⎦
   E **False**

16 A **False** enzyme induction
   B **True** increases plasma levels of phenobarbitone and phenytoin
   C **False** enzyme induction. Acute effects may produce enzyme inhibition
   D **True** inhibition of xanthine oxidase; increases blood levels of anticoagulants, uricosuric agents, 6-mercaptopurine and azathioprine
   E **True** inhibition of aldehyde dehydrogenase

17   Drug distribution throughout the body is influenced by
A   the lipid solubility of the drug
B   the pK of the drug
C   the plasma half-life of the drug
D   the presence of specific drug receptors
E   the extent of protein binding

18   Use of the following drugs should be avoided in late pregnancy because of adverse effects on the newborn
A   potassium iodide
B   benzyl penicillin
C   carbimazole
D   chloroquine
E   insulin

19   Drugs which produce a Coombs-positive haemolytic anaemia include
A   rifampicin
B   benzyl penicillin
C   isoniazid
D   co-trimoxazole
E   propranolol

20   In the treatment of hypertension
A   hydralazine can precipitate angina pectoris
B   methyldopa acts directly on arteriolar smooth muscle
C   debrisoquine produces ejaculatory failure
D   cardioselective beta-blockers are more effective in reducing blood pressure than are non-selective beta-blockers
E   thiazide diuretics aggravate the control of diabetes mellitus

21   Isoniazid therapy for active tuberculosis
A   produces a peripheral neuropathy
B   produces toxic effects more commonly in slow acetylators
C   should be used in combination with other antituberculosis drugs
D   readily crosses the blood–brain barrier after oral administration
E   produces cholestatic jaundice

17 A **True**   fat stores may act as drug reservoirs, e.g. thiopentone
    B **True**   weak bases are concentrated by the cells
    C **False** the half-life of a drug is determined by the volume of distribution and the elimination kinetics
    D **True**   beta-adrenergic blockers, digoxin, verapamil
    E **True**   sulphonamides are strongly protein-bound, limiting tissue penetration

18 A **True**   goitre, hypothyroidism or hyperthyroidism
    B **False** though safe, in utero sensitization may occur
    C **True**   goitre and hypothyroidism ◦
    D **False** risk of retinal damage is low so advantages outweigh the disadvantages
    E **False** neonatal hypoglycaemia can occur after delivery (but tight glycaemic control is required during labour). Drugs cross the placenta by simple diffusion; lipid-soluble, non-ionized drugs readily cross the placenta

19 A **True**   usually the immune complex of the drug and immunoglobulin attaches to the red blood cells. In contrast, penicillin binds directly to the red blood cells
    B **True**
    C **True**
    D **True**
    E **False**

20 A **True**   reduction in afterload causes reflex tachycardia
    B **False** methyldopa acts as a false neurotransmitter in adrenergic neurones within the CNS
    C **True**   acts as a sympathetic ganglion blocker
    D **False** hypotensive effect is unrelated to β_2 receptor effects
    E **True**   inhibition of peripheral glucose utilization

21 A **True**   isoniazid toxicity is usually related to dose and acetylator status. The possibility of neuropathy may be reduced with concomitant pyridoxine therapy since the drug interferes with pyridoxine metabolism
    B **True**
    C **True**   the possibility of inducing bacterial resistance makes multiple therapy mandatory
    D **True**   pyrazinamide and isoniazid are the two antituberculosis drugs which most readily penetrate the CSF
    E **False** it is hepatocellular jaundice that might occur

22   Drugs which impair the efficacy of oral contraception include
   A   phenytoin
   B   digoxin
   C   rifampicin
   D   salbutamol
   E   ampicillin

23   In the treatment of angina pectoris
   A   nitrates act by reducing the venous return
   B   cardioselective beta-blockers are more effective than non-cardioselective beta-blockers
   C   tolerance is less likely with transdermal nitrate therapy
   D   calcium-channel blockers diminish coronary vascular tone
   E   beta-blockade prevents the tachycardia induced by nitrates

24   A grey-blue discoloration of the mucous membranes is a recognized finding in chronic poisoning with
   A   mercury
   B   lead
   C   bismuth
   D   silver
   E   gold

25   Signs of chronic lead poisoning include
   A   encephalopathy
   B   abdominal colic
   C   microcytic, hypochromic anaemia
   D   gout
   E   motor neuropathy and wrist-drop

26   Following intentional drug overdosage
   A   recent alcohol consumption is often involved
   B   a previous history of drug overdosage is unusual
   C   most patients readily admit to suicidal intent
   D   serious suicidal intent should be suspected in alcoholics
   E   serious suicidal intent is commoner in females

22 A **True**   enzyme induction and accelerated metabolism
   B **False**
   C **True**   enzyme induction and accelerated metabolism
   D **False**
   E **True**   displacement from protein binding increases drug
               clearance and effects on bowel flora accelerate
               enterohepatic elimination

23 A **True**   their main effect, although nitrates are also coronary
               vasodilators
   B **False** metoprolol and atenolol are no more effective than
               propranolol but are less likely to produce
               bronchospasm
   C **False** it is more of a problem and can be managed by
               removal of patches for 2 or 3 hours in 24 hours
   D **True**   particularly nifedipine
   E **True**   hence the usefulness of combining these agents

24 A **True**   most heavy metal poisonings produce a similar
               clinical syndrome, with skin, cerebral, renal and
               gastrointestinal features. Chloroquine also produces
               buccal pigmentation
   B **True**
   C **True**
   D **True**
   E **True**

25 A **True**   usually associated with very high blood lead levels
   B **True**   metallic taste in the mouth and colic are the earliest
               features
   C **True**   more common in children; basophilic stippling is the
               commoner finding in adults
   D **True**   saturnine gout due to renal insufficiency
   E **True**   muscle weakness is greater in the forearm extensors;
               motor neuropathy is more common than sensory
               neuropathy

26 A **True**   50% have recently consumed alcohol and the clinical
               features are accordingly altered
   B **False** at least 50% of such patients have a history of
               multiple drug overdosages
   C **False** only a minority express suicidal intent
   D **True**   males and alcoholic patients are at greater risk of
               eventual suicide
   E **False**

27   The clinical features of acute iron poisoning include
A   burns around the mouth
B   peripheral cyanosis
C   haematemesis
D   drowsiness
E   thrombocytopenia

28   Oral corticosteroid therapy should be avoided in the presence of
A   acute gout
B   systemic hypertension
C   herpes zoster
D   herpes simplex keratitis
E   active duodenal ulceration

29   Pethidine
A   is suitable for the relief of chronic pain in terminal care
B   relaxes ureteric spasm in renal colic
C   is less likely to cause addiction than morphine
D   is less likely to cause respiratory depression than morphine
E   causes delayed gastric emptying

30   Benzyl penicillin
A   is destroyed by gastric acid
B   is the drug of first choice in beta-haemolytic streptococcal
    infections
C   produces convulsions in overdosage
D   is effective against beta-lactamase-producing organisms
E   should be given intrathecally in bacterial meningitis

31   Complications of acute ethyl alcohol intoxication include
A   hypoglycaemia
B   lactic acidosis
C   hyponatraemia
D   left ventricular failure
E   false-localizing neurological signs

27	A	**False**	strong acid and alkali solutions will produce corrosive mouth changes
	B	**True**	circulatory collapse and metabolic acidosis may occur within 4 hours or be delayed for 12–24 hours
	C	**True**	haemorrhagic gastroenteritis is common, resulting in vomiting, diarrhoea, abdominal pain and gastrointestinal bleeding
	D	**True**	lassitude and drowsiness indicate serious poisoning with impending encephalopathy
	E	**False**	

28	A	**False**	acute gout may respond dramatically to corticosteroid therapy
	B	**True**	sodium retention promotes hypertension
	C	**True**	disseminated varicella can occur
	D	**True**	corneal ulceration may progress rapidly
	E	**True**	the effect is weak; benefit of enteric-coated medication is speculative

29	A	**False**	unsuitable due to its short duration of action
	B	**False**	ureteric muscle contraction may increase despite pain relief
	C	**False**	approximately similar dependence potential
	D	**False**	equipotent in the production of respiratory depression
	E	**True**	all opioids delay gastric emptying

30	A	**True**	phenoxymethyl penicillin is acid-stable and can be administered orally
	B	**True**	relatively ineffective against enterococci – less so
	C	**True**	rarely encountered except in renal failure
	D	**False**	90% of hospital staphylococci are resistant due to beta-lactamase activity
	E	**False**	CSF penetration is sufficient; intrathecal administration is hazardous

31	A	**True**	due to the impaired peripheral glucose uptake, hyperinsulinism and an inhibition of gluconeogenesis, diabetics are at special risk
	B	**True**	by the inhibition of hepatic lactate uptake and gluconeogenesis from lactate
	C	**True**	inhibits the secretion of antidiuretic hormone promoting a diuresis. The resulting thirst may produce water intoxication when the diuretic effect ceases
	D	**False**	chronic alcohol abuse may produce a congestive cardiomyopathy
	E	**True**	coma, respiratory depression, unequal pupil diameters, strabismus and nystagmus

32   In acute methyl alcohol poisoning
A   the agent is poorly absorbed from the small bowel
B   the agent is excreted in the urine unchanged
C   the treatment of choice is ethyl alcohol
D   metabolic acidosis commonly occurs
E   blindness results if treatment is delayed

33   Digoxin is likely to be useful in the treatment of
A   thyrotoxic atrial fibrillation
B   ventricular tachycardia
C   hypertrophic obstructive cardiomyopathy
D   atrial flutter with 2:1 block
E   re-entrant tachycardia in Wolff–Parkinson–White syndrome

34   Cytotoxic agents which act as pyrimidine antagonists include
A   thioguanine
B   methotrexate
C   vinblastine
D   cytarabine
E   cisplatin

35   Characteristic features of severe paracetamol poisoning include
A   hypoglycaemia
B   acute renal failure
C   hypotension
D   delirium
E   hyperpyrexia

36   Dilated pupils are a recognized finding in acute poisoning with
A   phenytoin
B   theophylline
C   imipramine
D   chlorpromazine
E   carbon monoxide

37   Co-trimoxazole is an appropriate antibiotic choice in the management of
A   typhoid carriers
B   gas gangrene
C   gonorrhoea
D   prostatitis
E   *Pneumocystis carinii* infection

32	A	False	well absorbed and oxidized to formaldehyde and formic acid in the liver and kidneys
	B	False	
	C	True	ethyl alcohol retards the oxidation of methanol
	D	True	requiring intravenous fluid and alkali therapy. Haemodialysis may be indicated
	E	True	early treatment with ethyl alcohol should prevent blindness which is due to the effect of formaldehyde on the retinal cells

33	A	False	inability to control ventricular rate in patient with atrial fibrillation may be the first feature of thyrotoxicosis
	B	False	
	C	False	of no proven benefit and potentially hazardous
	D	True	slows A/V conduction
	E	False	potentially dangerous as it may paradoxically increase anomalous conduction

34	A	False	interferes with purine biosynthesis
	B	True	dihydrofolate reductase inhibitor, so affects purines and pyrimidines
	C	False	interferes with microtubule assembly, causing metaphase arrest
	D	True	
	E	False	an alkylating agent

35	A	True	
	B	True	with or without liver toxicity
	C	True	
	D	False	not enough to be clinically significant
	E	False	

36	A	False	nystagmus is the usual eye sign
	B	True	a sympathetic effect
	C	True	an anticholinergic effect
	D	True	
	E	False	papilloedema is the usual eye sign

37	A	True	
	B	False	
	C	False	
	D	True	and epididymo-orchitis
	E	True	high doses required

BMF

only PCP indicated

38   Antibiotics which are safe to prescribe in renal failure include
- **A** tetracycline
- **B** clindamycin
- **C** cefotaxime
- **D** ampicillin
- **E** trimethoprim

39   Characteristic features of poisoning with organophosphorous insecticides include
- **A** dilated pupils
- **B** bradycardia
- **C** hypersalivation
- **D** pulmonary oedema
- **E** muscle fasciculation

40   Under International Olympic Committee rules a competing athlete developing headache and cough would be permitted to take
- **A** paracetamol
- **B** phenylpropanolamine
- **C** co-proxamol
- **D** pseudoephedrine
- **E** mefenamic acid

41   Zidovudine
- **A** is of proven benefit in HIV seroconversion syndromes
- **B** is metabolized principally in the liver
- **C** after conversion to zidovudine triphosphate inhibits HIV reverse transcriptase
- **D** slows the progression of clinical disease in asymptomatic HIV infection
- **E** reduces infectivity of HIV infected individuals

42   In the treatment of paracetamol poisoning
- **A** gastric lavage is useful up to 12 hours after the overdose
- **B** intravenous acetylcysteine is ineffective after 8 hours have elapsed since overdose
- **C** liver transplantation for acute hepatic failure is contraindicated
- **D** oral methionine is reserved for those presenting after 16 hours
- **E** wheeze is a recognized side-effect of acetylcysteine infusion

38 A **False** has anti-anabolic effect and can increase plasma urea
    B **True**
    C **True** half dose usually required
    D **True** dose may need to be reduced. Rashes more common
    E **True** smaller dose sometimes required

39 A **False** cholinesterase inhibition produces small pupils
    B **True** ⎫
    C **True** ⎬ cholinergic effects
    D **True** ⎭
    E **True**

40 A **True**
    B **False** nasal decongestants often contain banned sympathomimetic agents
    C **False** contains dextropropoxyphene—an opioid
    D **False**
    E **True**

41 A **False** but may give symptomatic relief in some patients with neuropathy
    B **True** 60–80% by glucuronidation
    C **True** prevents viral replication in newly infected cells
    D **False** no long-term benefit
    E **False**

42 A **False** gastric lavage useful up to 4 hours after event unless concomitant aspirin ingestion is suspected
    B **False** can be used up to 24 hours after event especially if patients encephalopathic
    C **False** specialist advice should be sought
    D **False**
    E **True** this is a pseudo-allergic reaction

43   In the use of anti-arrhythmic drug therapy
- A   mexiletine is a class Ib anti-arrhythmic agent and delays the depolarization phase
- B   adenosine is indicated in ventricular tachycardia
- C   amiodarone is a class III anti-arrhythmic agent prolonging the duration of the action potential
- D   verapamil is a class II anti-arrhythmic agent and inhibits the fast sodium channel
- E   phenytoin accelerates conduction in Purkinje fibres

44   In the treatment of acute left ventricular failure
- A   frusemide acts immediately by reducing afterload
- B   nitrate therapy is hazardous in severe mitral stenosis
- C   quinidine therapy enhances the renal clearance of digoxin
- D   hydralazine increases the severity of mitral regurgitation
- E   aminophylline is best avoided in acute myocardial infarction

45   Bromocriptine therapy
- A   increases dopaminergic neurone activity in the CNS
- B   produces nausea, vomiting and weight loss
- C   is contraindicated in hypertensive patients
- D   usefully reduces pituitary tumour size in acromegaly
- E   is the treatment of choice in pituitary microprolactinomas

46   Captopril therapy
- A   is best reserved for severe heart failure
- B   often results in irritating cough
- C   produces renal failure in bilateral renal artery stenosis
- D   is contraindicated in pregnancy hypertension
- E   causes hypokalaemia

43 A **True**   orally effective and not as rapidly metabolized as
                lignocaine
   B **False** is very useful in supraventricular tachycardias,
                including those associated with accessory pathways
   C **True**   long half-life (30 days); useful in WPW syndrome.
                Side-effects include thyroid dysfunction,
                photosensitization and corneal deposits
   D **False** class IV agent inhibiting the slow calcium channel.
                Beta-blockers are class II agents and class I agents
                inhibit the fast sodium channel
   E **True**   especially useful in ventricular arrhythmias
                associated with digoxin or hypokalaemia

44 A **True**   rapid reduction in pulmonary arterial pressure
                occurs before the diuresis begins
   B **True**   low cardiac output states are a relative
                contraindication because of pre-load reduction and
                the need for high filling pressures
   C **False** caution is required because of impaired renal
                clearance of digoxin
   D **False** afterload reduction improves LV output thus
                reducing mitral regurgitation
   E **True**   increased likelihood of ventricular arrhythmias

45 A **True**   useful in the treatment of parkinsonism and
                hyperprolactinaemia
   B **True**   therapy should commence at low dosage
   C **False** postural hypotension may be avoided by starting at
                low dosage
   D **False** little effect on tumour size but will reduce growth
                hormone
   E **True**   treatment of choice in microprolactinomas;
                suprasellar extension and erosion of the sella are
                indications for surgical assessment

46 A **False** beneficial effect has been shown in asymptomatic LV
                impairment
   B **True**   a common side-effect which resolves when drug is
                stopped
   C **True**   bilateral renal artery stenosis is often unmasked
   D **True**   significant fetal risk
   E **False** may produce hyperkalaemia by lowering
                aldosterone levels

47 Drugs which are safe to prescribe in breast-feeding mothers include
- A salazopyrine
- B lithium carbonate
- C oxytetracycline
- D propranolol
- E mefloquine

48 Treatment with misoprostol
- A is contraindicated in pregnant women
- B increases the rate of healing of gastric ulcers associated with non-steroidal anti-inflammatory drug (NSAID) therapy
- C produces abdominal pain and diarrhoea
- D inhibits gastric acid secretion
- E is mandatory in elderly patients using NSAIDs

49 Useful treatments in the management of vomiting induced by cytotoxic agents include
- A ondansetron
- B domperidone
- C lorazepam
- D nabilone
- E metoclopramide

50 Recognized side-effects of cyclosporin therapy include
- A hypomagnesaemia
- B hypertrichosis
- C pulmonary infiltrates
- D avascular necrosis
- E convulsions

47	A	**True**	safe in modest dosages
	B	**False**	serious side-effects have been reported
	C	**False**	chelating effects of calcium in milk reduce the risk of discoloration of teeth, but the drug is best avoided
	D	**True**	
	E	**False**	should be avoided in pregnancy and for 3 months after

48	A	**True**	increases uterine contractility and may cause miscarriage
	B	**True**	one of its principal indications
	C	**True**	the commonest side-effect
	D	**True**	as well as cytoprotective properties
	E	**False**	better to withdraw NSAIDs if dyspepsia occurs

49	A	**True**	$5HT_3$ receptor antagonist
	B	**True**	dopaminergic receptor antagonist
	C	**True**	has been shown to have some benefit
	D	**True**	this semi-synthetic cannabinoid has more side-effects in the elderly
	E	**True**	dopaminergic receptor antagonist often combined with dexamethasone therapy

50	A	**True**	
	B	**True**	
	C	**False**	reported with azathioprine
	D	**False**	is usually the result of concomitant corticosteroid therapy
	E	**True**	

Cardiology

1 **In patients with hyperlipoproteinaemia**
   A the children of patients with familial type 11a hyperlipoproteinaemia have a 50% chance of inheriting the trait
   B chylomicrons consist primarily of triglycerides
   C plasma cholesterol is reduced in the nephrotic syndrome
   D long-term gemfibrozil therapy decreases the incidence of cardiac events
   E plasma cholesterol decreases with age

2 **In infective endocarditis**
   A alpha-haemolytic streptococci are the commonest causative organisms
   B prophylactic tetracycline therapy is indicated prior to dental extraction
   C diffuse glomerulonephritis leads to irreversible renal failure
   D valve replacement is contraindicated until after at least 2 weeks of antibiotic therapy
   E blood cultures are best taken during peaks of pyrexia

3 **Aortic incompetence**
   A is associated with a bicuspid aortic valve
   B causes 'pistol-shot' sounds at the femoral arteries
   C causes capillary pulsation visible in the nail bed
   D can result from type B (De Bakey III) aortic dissection
   E has a severity which is proportional to the intensity of the diastolic murmur

4 **Chest pain is likely to be due to angina pectoris if**
   A it occurs consistently at the beginning of exercise but wears off as exercise continues
   B hyperventilation causes T wave inversion on the ECG
   C exercise testing shows ST depression with a rapid up-slope
   D glyceryl trinitrate relieves the pain within 5 minutes
   E exercise reduces the left ventricular ejection fraction

1 A **True**   autosomal dominant
   B **True**
   C **False**   the nephrotic syndrome increases cholesterol and
                  triglyceride concentration
   D **True**   but does not prolong life
   E **False**   increases progressively with age

2 A **True**   in 50% of cases, the organism arises from mouth or
                  oropharynx
   B **False**   not bactericidal; benzyl penicillin, amoxycillin or
                  erythromycin should be used
   C **False**   renal failure reverses with treatment of endocarditis
   D **False**   valve replacement is indicated at all stages of
                  treatment if heart failure supervenes
   E **False**   timing blood cultures with peaks of pyrexia does not
                  significantly increase the yield of positive cultures;
                  six to eight samples should be taken in the first 24
                  hours

3 A **True**   stenosis is more common
   B **True**
   C **True**
   D **False**   involves the descending aorta only
   E **False**   there is no good correlation between intensity of
                  murmur and severity of incompetence

4 A **True**   'first-effort' angina
   B **False**   hyperventilation induces T wave changes in health
   C **False**   an ischaemic ST segment shift is down-sloping,
                  horizontal or of the 'slow-rising' type
   D **True**
   E **True**

5 Aortic stenosis
  A in some patients is asymptomatic even when severe
  B causes fixed splitting of the second heart sound
  C produces a thrill in the suprasternal notch
  D is unlikely to be severe if the ECG is normal
  E is unlikely to be severe if the blood pressure is normal

6 Ventricular fibrillation is a recognized hazard in
  A ventricular ectopics occurring on the peak of the R wave
  B digoxin toxicity
  C prolonged QT interval
  D complete (third-degree) heart block
  E overdrive pacing

7 Tricuspid incompetence
  A causes giant 'a' waves in the neck veins
  B causes hepatic pulsation
  C is usually secondary to right ventricular dilatation
  D commonly causes pulmonary embolism
  E has a murmur which decreases with inspiration

8 In hypertension
  A ECG changes of left ventricular hypertrophy improve with
     lowering of blood pressure
  B treatment with prazosin unmasks diabetes mellitus
  C anxiety increases the pulse pressure but does not increase
     the systolic pressure
  D salt restriction lowers blood pressure in most individuals
  E hypertension is aggravated by oestrogen therapy

9 Infective endocarditis is associated with
  A arthralgias
  B ostium secundum rather than ostium primum atrial septal
     defect
  C normal leucocyte count
  D haematuria
  E negative blood cultures

5 A **True**
   B **False**   reversed splitting or a single second heart sound but
                   not fixed splitting
   C **True**   often felt better at the suprasternal notch rather than
                   at the aortic area of the chest wall
   D **True**
   E **False**   blood pressure is an unreliable guide. The pulse
                   characteristics are a better guide

6 A **False**   the 'vulnerable period' for ventricular ectopics is
                   near the peak of the T̲ wave
   B **True**   shortens the refractory period of cardiac muscle
   C **True**   increased likelihood of R on T ectopics and increased
                   excitability (torsades de pointes)
   D **True**   transient ventricular fibrillation can be present
                   during a Stokes–Adams attack in a patient with
                   complete heart block
   E **False**   pacing the ventricle at a faster rate can prevent
                   attacks of ventricular tachycardia and fibrillation

7 A **False**   'CV' waves are seen due to rise in right atrial
                   pressure during ventricular systole
   B **True**
   C **True**
   D **False**
   E **False**   characteristically increases with inspiration

8 A **True**
   B **False**   alpha-adrenergic blockers have no effect on blood
                   sugar
   C **False**   both are increased
   D **True**   rarely sufficient to provide the sole therapy for
                   hypertension
   E **True**

9 A **True**
   B **False**   the lack of turbulent flow makes the defect resistant
                   to endocarditis
   C **True**
   D **True**   focal glomerulonephritis and septic emboli
   E **True**   10–20% are culture-negative

10   Characteristic features of sick sinus syndrome include
  A   an increased incidence of cerebral embolism
  B   association with coronary artery disease in young patients
  C   atrial tachyarrhythmias
  D   a prolongation of the sinus node recovery time
  E   endocardial pacing improving life expectancy

11   Atrial arrhythmias are a recognized complication of
  A   digoxin toxicity
  B   mitral valve prolapse
  C   Lown–Ganong–Levine syndrome
  D   lobar pneumonia
  E   verapamil therapy

12   Coarctation of the aorta in adults is associated with
  A   a vascular constriction which is often proximal to the left
       subclavian artery
  B   a higher incidence of aortic stenosis
  C   Marfan's syndrome
  D   a to-and-fro continuous murmur
  E   an increased risk of cerebrovascular accidents

13   In the electrocardiogram
  A   hypokalaemia produces flattened T waves
  B   right ventricular hypertrophy causes clockwise rotation
  C   pathological Q waves are usually the first sign of infarction
  D   a QT interval of 500 milliseconds is normal
  E   Mobitz type II atrioventricular block does not show
       progressive lengthening of the PR interval

**14   A poorer prognosis after acute myocardial infarction is
associated with**
  A   transient pulmonary oedema
  B   ventricular fibrillation within 12 hours of onset of infarction
  C   left ventricular ejection fraction in range 20–30%
  D   patients aged 75 or over
  E   inferior rather than an anterior infarction

15   In the PA chest X-ray, the cardiac silhouette
  A   accurately identifies left atrial size
  B   is usually increased in size in right ventricular hypertrophy
  C   is within normal limits in chronic hypoadrenalism
  D   correlates with the severity of hypertensive heart disease
  E   shows a prominent pulmonary artery shadow in normal
       adolescents.

10	A	**True**	anticoagulant therapy may be indicated
	B	**False**	sino-atrial disease in young patients is usually not due to coronary disease
	C	**True**	the tachycardia/bradycardia syndrome is a form of sino-atrial disease
	D	**True**	
	E	**False**	pacing is for symptomatic benefit

11	A	**True**	digoxin can cause any arrhythmia
	B	**True**	
	C	**True**	accessory pathway produces a re-entry tachycardia
	D	**True**	
	E	**False**	used to treat atrial arrhythmias

12	A	**False**	just distal to the left subclavian artery
	B	**True**	and aortic dissection
	C	**False**	but also causes aortic dissection
	D	**False**	systolic murmur only
	E	**True**	due to hypertension, atheroma, dissection and berry aneurysms

13	A	**True**	also seen in hypercalcaemia
	B	**True**	
	C	**False**	ST elevation is usually seen first
	D	**False**	the normal QT is less than 440 msec and is rate dependent
	E	**True**	Mobitz type I (Wenckebach) block has a lengthening of the PR interval; Mobitz type II has a fixed PR interval

14	A	**True**	
	B	**False**	late ventricular fibrillation is a bad prognostic sign
	C	**True**	
	D	**True**	coexisting diseases are more common, e.g. diabetes
	E	**False**	inferior infarcts tend to cause less damage and have a better prognosis

15	A	**False**	can reveal left atrial enlargement but not accurately quantify the size: echocardiography is much better
	B	**False**	the right ventricle lies within the cardiac silhouette
	C	**True**	
	D	**True**	
	E	**True**	

16   M-mode echocardiography reliably detects the presence of
A   right coronary artery stenosis
B   mild mitral stenosis
C   hypertrophic cardiomyopathy
D   mild mitral reflux
E   Libman–Sacks endocarditis

17   In invasive cardiac investigation
A   a gradient of 30 mmHg across the aortic valve usually indicates severe stenosis
B   pulmonary artery oxygen saturation is independent of the cardiac output
C   the mortality from coronary angiography is approximately 5%
D   in constrictive pericarditis the end-diastolic pressures are equal in both ventricles
E   a left ventricular end-diastolic pressure of 25 mmHg indicates a myocardial abnormality in the absence of valve disease

18   After mitral valve replacement for mitral regurgitation
A   the patient is no longer at risk from endocarditis
B   the left atrial size returns to normal
C   X-ray screening is useful in assessing post-operative valve function
D   a reduction in intensity of valve clicks is of little significance
E   concomitant ranitidine therapy reduces the efficacy of warfarin

19   In atrial tachyarrhythmias
A   the delta wave in Wolff–Parkinson–White syndrome is due to myocardial activation via an additional conduction pathway
B   atrial pacing can control atrial tachycardias
C   atrial fibrillation is a recognized complication of the Wolff–Parkinson–White syndrome
D   polyuria suggests a ventricular rather than supraventricular focus
E   atrial tachycardias usually arise from a re-entry mechanism when the ECG is otherwise normal

16 A **False** proximal left coronary artery disease can sometimes
be seen
    B **True**
    C **True**
    D **False** Doppler ultrasound is more helpful
    E **False** the vegetations are usually too small

17 A **False** gradients greater than 50 mmHg
    B **False** pulmonary artery oxygen saturation reflects cardiac
output as the arterio-venous oxygen saturation
difference increases as cardiac output falls
    C **False** 0.1–0.2% mortality
    D **True**
    E **True**

18 A **False** patients with prosthetic valves are particularly
vulnerable to endocarditis
    B **False**
    C **True** for prosthetic valves with a tilting disc or a ball
    D **False** indicates thrombus developing at the valve
    E **False** interaction with warfarin and cimetidine

19 A **True** accessory pathway of Kent
    B **True**
    C **True** occurs in about 15% of patients
    D **False** possibly as a result of atrial natriuretic peptide
release
    E **True**

20   Characteristic features of severe mitral stenosis include
  A   a sternal heave
  B   a loud third heart sound
  C   no audible diastolic murmur
  D   ascites
  E   a mean left atrial pressure of 15 mmHg

21   In mitral incompetence
  A   due to mitral valve prolapse, the murmur is unaffected by respiration or posture
  B   the murmur often radiates to the base when the posterior cusp is abnormal
  C   the severity is best assessed by pulmonary wedge pressure studies
  D   a loud third heart sound is common if the incompetence is severe
  E   congenital endocardial cushion defects are a recognized predisposing factor

22   In acute pericarditis
  A   pain radiates to the shoulders and back
  B   due to recent myocardial infarction, steroid therapy should be given
  C   anticoagulants are contraindicated
  D   pain is unaffected by posture
  E   echocardiography will demonstrate a small pericardial effusion

23   In congenital ventricular septal defects
  A   with Eisenmenger syndrome there is a left-to-right shunt
  B   small defects usually close spontaneously
  C   if endocarditis develops the left ventricular cavity is usually involved
  D   the murmur radiates to the carotids
  E   the defect typically involves the membranous part of the septum

24   In the normal heart
  A   the sinus node is situated in the inter-atrial septum
  B   the coronary sinus orifice opens into the right ventricle
  C   the foramen ovale is rarely patent after the first year of life
  D   the mitral anterior cusp is larger than the posterior cusp
  E   the right coronary artery usually supplies the inferior surface of the left ventricle

20 A **True**   due to enlargement of the right ventricle
    B **False**   impaired diastolic filling prevents a third heart sound
    C **True**   'murmurless' mitral stenosis occurs when the
                   cardiac output is low
    D **True**   due to right heart failure
    E **False**   left atrial pressure is markedly elevated (normal ≤ 13
                   mmHg)

21 A **False**
    B **True**
    C **False**   radionuclide ventriculography or angiography
    D **True**   due to rapid re-entry of blood in early diastole
    E **True**

22 A **True**
    B **False**   non-steroidal anti-inflammatory drugs are better,
                   although steroids often required for post-MI
                   syndrome
    C **True**   due to the risk of a haemopericardium
    D **False**   characteristically, posture affects the pain
    E **True**   the best method

23 A **False**   right to left
    B **True**
    C **False**   the 'jet lesion' occurs on the right ventricle
    D **False**   localized to the left sternal edge and associated with
                   a palpable thrill
    E **True**

24 A **False**   near the superior vena cava
    B **False**   right atrium
    C **False**   'probe-patent' in a third of normal adults
    D **True**
    E **True**

25 In dissection of the aorta
- A aortic incompetence is common
- B the pain increases gradually over several hours
- C it is essential to identify the re-entry site of the dissection by angiography
- D CT scanning of thorax is helpful in the diagnosis
- E urgent surgical correction is necessary in type B (de Bakey III)

26 In rheumatic fever
- A there is an antecedent history of group A beta-haemolytic streptococcal infection
- B a short rumbling diastolic murmur indicates mitral valvitis
- C erythema marginatum characteristically spares the face
- D the ESR is usually elevated
- E small-joint rather than large-joint arthropathy is typical

27 In chronic constrictive pericarditis
- A paroxysmal nocturnal dyspnoea is characteristic
- B irradiation of the thorax is a recognized cause
- C ascites and splenomegaly are typical features
- D right and left ventricular end diastolic pressures are equal
- E a high venous pressure with rapid X descent is typical

28 In the treatment of chronic biventricular cardiac failure
- A treatment with enalapril prolongs survival
- B nitrates usefully decrease afterload
- C cardiac transplantation is of proven benefit
- D digoxin is most useful when associated with atrial fibrillation
- E bedrest produces a significant diuresis

29 In considering the insertion of a permanent cardiac pacemaker
- A DDD is optimal for atrial fibrillation with atrioventricular block
- B asymptomatic pauses of less than 2 seconds on Holter monitoring merit a VVI pacemaker
- C dual-chamber pacing is useful when left ventricular function is poor
- D VVI are more likely than DDD pacemakers to produce the pacemaker syndrome
- E sinus node disease with normal AV conduction merit AAI pacemakers

25 A **True**
    B **False**   usually maximal from the onset
    C **False**   surgical treatment is directed to the area of the proximal tear
    D **True**
    E **False**   usually treated medically initially

26 A **True**   usually within 3–4 weeks prior to onset
    B **True**
    C **True**   unlike SLE or adult Still's disease
    D **True**
    E **False**

27 A **False**   right ventricular failure is much more prominent than left
    B **True**
    C **True**
    D **True**
    E **False**   sudden brief filling of right ventricle produces a typically prominent 'y' descent $\left(x r y \right)$.
                    x ry.

28 A **True**
    B **False**   nitrates reduce pre-load
    C **True**   this treatment limited by donor numbers
    D **True**
    E **True**   increases renal perfusion

29 A **False**   VVI with adaptive rate pacing is better
    B **False**   insufficient evidence of disturbance
    C **True**   atrial contribution to ventricular filling is important
    D **True**   VVI = ventricular pacing; ventricular sensing; inhibited by host signal
    E **True**   ideally single chamber atrial adaptive rate pacing

30   Significant risk factors for the development of ischaemic heart disease include
A   elevated plasma HDL-cholesterol concentration
B   family history of type 2 diabetes
C   low factor VIIIc plasma concentration
D   obsessional personality
E   smoking five cigarettes daily for 10 years

31   Recognized causes of congestive cardiomyopathy include
A   polymyositis
B   alcohol abuse
C   endomyocardial fibrosis
D   transfusion haemosiderosis
E   Friedreich's ataxia

32   In hypertrophic obstructive cardiomyopathy (HOCM)
A   24-hour ambulatory ECG monitoring is useful to identify non-sustained ventricular tachycardia
B   abnormality of the β cardiac myosin heavy-chain gene is a recognized finding
C   the ejection fraction is characteristically low
D   abnormal systolic motion of the mitral valve is seen echocardiographically
E   the right ventricle is uninvolved

33   Raynaud's phenomenon is a recognized feature of
A   thromboangiitis obliterans
B   renal carcinoma
C   diabetic sensory neuropathy
D   systemic sclerosis
E   giant-cell arteritis

34   Pulmonary hypertension due to increased pulmonary blood flow is characteristic of
A   chronic bronchitis and emphysema
B   mitral stenosis
C   multiple pulmonary emboli
D   persistent ductus arteriosus
E   ostium primum atrial septal defect

30 A **False** a low HDL-cholesterol is of greater risk
   B **True**
   C **False**
   D **False**
   E **True**

31 A **True** rarely affects cardiac muscle
   B **True**
   C **False** causes restrictive cardiomyopathy
   D **True** also haemochromatosis
   E **True**

32 A **True** thus amiodarone treatment may confer some benefit
   B **True**
   C **False** small LV cavity but normal ejection fraction
   D **True**
   E **False** both sides involved, the right less markedly so

33 A **True** arteriosclerotic arterial disease
   B **True**
   C **False** skin blood flow may be increased due to sympathetic denervation
   D **True**
   E **True**

34 A **False** hypoxia causes pulmonary vasoconstriction and increases pulmonary vascular resistance
   B **False** } increased vascular resistance
   C **False** }
   D **True**
   E **True**

35   In deep venous thrombosis

- A   most patients have ankle oedema
- B   pyrexia is typically the only sign of pulmonary embolism developing post-operatively
- C   venography is the best diagnostic test
- D   occult malignancy should be suspected if no obvious predisposing factor is found
- E   treatment with warfarin should be life long

36   Coronary artery by-pass surgery is of proven benefit in

- A   asymptomatic patients with abnormal exercise ECGs
- B   left main coronary stenosis in symptomatic patients
- C   symptomatic patients despite maximal anti-anginal therapy
- D   triple vessel disease in patients with impaired left ventricular function
- E   symptomatic patients with normal coronary angiography

37   Useful treatments in the management of unstable angina include

- A   aspirin in dose of 150 mg/day
- B   subcutaneous low-molecular-weight heparin
- C   intravenous isosorbide mononitrate
- D   atenolol therapy
- E   diazepam therapy

38   In deep inspiration

- A   the murmur of ventricular septal defect becomes louder
- B   reverse splitting of second heart sound develops in pulmonary hypertension
- C   the murmur of tricuspid stenosis becomes louder
- D   blood pressure falls in pericardial constriction
- E   the opening snap in mitral stenosis is louder

39   Palpitation is a recognized feature of

- A   excessive coffee drinking
- B   nebulized bronchodilator treatment
- C   hypoglycaemia
- D   carcinoid syndrome
- E   Wolff–Parkinson–White syndrome

35 A **False** many patients have no symptoms or signs
    B **True**
    C **True** although Doppler ultrasound velocity profiles useful for veins above knee
    D **True** also consider anti-cardiolipin syndrome and alcohol abuse
    E **False** unless recurrent episodes, treatment is usually for no more than 3 months

36 A **False**
    B **True** prolongs survival
    C **True** alleviates symptoms
    D **True** a good indication for surgery
    E **False** risk of surgery is greater than the risk from variant angina

37 A **True**
    B **True**
    C **True**
    D **True**
    E **False**

38 A **False** respiration has little effect
    B **False** in hypertrophic obstructive cardiomyopathy, left bundle branch block and aortic stenosis
    C **True**
    D **True**
    E **False**

39 A **True**
    B **True**
    C **True**
    D **True**
    E **True**

40 The following are usually of no clinical significance when found during ambulatory ECG monitoring
   A   infrequent ventricular extrasystoles
   B   first-degree heart block
   C   Mobitz type II atrioventricular (AV) block
   D   ventricular tachycardia
   E   brief paroxysms of atrial fibrillation

40 A **True**
   B **True**   common in young people or athletes with high vagal
                    tone
   C **False**
   D **False** ⎫ requires further assessment
   E **False** ⎭

Gastroenterology

1 Aphthous ulceration of the mouth is a typical feature of
   A Addisonian pernicious anaemia
   B gluten-sensitive enteropathy
   C iron-deficiency anaemia
   D Reiter's syndrome
   E Crohn's disease

2 A 55-year-old woman with a 15-year history of heartburn
   presents with 3 months of progressive dysphagia, initially for
   solids and more recently for liquids and has lost 10 kg in weight
   A the likeliest diagnosis is achalasia
   B the picture suggests severe ulcerative oesophagitis
   C a normal barium meal obviates the need for endoscopy
   D in view of the short history of dysphagia an early resectable
      oesophageal carcinoma is likely
   E the 5-year survival rate of oesophageal carcinoma is less than
      20%

3 Recognized features of coeliac disease include
   A an increased incidence of circulating antireticulin antibodies
   B a clinical response to corticosteroid therapy
   C hypersplenism
   D a reduction in the circulating T-cell population
   E intolerance to maize products

4 Findings of diagnostic significance on rectal biopsy occur in
   A amoebiasis
   B giardiasis
   C Crohn's disease
   D schistosomiasis
   E lymphogranuloma venereum

1 A **False** buccal pigmentation
   B **True**
   C **False**   less common in iron than folate deficiency
   D **True**
   E **True**   may be sole presentation

2 A **False**   the story suggests an oesophageal carcinoma
   B **False**   and this should be regarded as oesophageal
                  carcinoma until proved otherwise
   C **False**   radiology is often helpful, but endoscopy and biopsy
                  will be required
   D **False**   symptoms occur late when the diameter of the
                  oesophageal lumen is reduced by at least 50%; 80%
                  have lymph node involvement at presentation
   E **True**

3 A **True**   circulating immune complexes may also be detected
   B **True**   this is one of the arguments in support of the
                 hypothesis that coeliac disease has an
                 immunological basis
   C **False**   splenic atrophy occurs with Howell–Jolly bodies on
                  the blood film
   D **True**
   E **False**   the toxic factor is alpha-1 gliadin, which is found in
                  wheat, rye, barley and possibly oats, but not in rice or
                  maize

4 A **True**   cysts may be identified either in rectal biopsies or in
                 associated mucus
   B **False**   the diagnosis is made on small-intestinal biopsies or
                  by the identification of cysts in the faeces
   C **True**   a granuloma in the rectal biopsy is diagnostic of
                 Crohn's disease in the presence of other features of
                 inflammatory bowel disease
   D **True**   the ova may be seen in an inflammatory reaction in
                 mucosa or submucosa
   E **False**   the findings on rectal biopsy are those of a chronic
                  non-specific proctitis

5   In chronic liver disease
    A propranolol increases portal venous pressure
    B congenital hepatic fibrosis is associated with renal tubular acidosis
    C gynaecomastia is associated with elevated serum oestradiol concentrations
    D functional renal failure (hepatorenal syndrome) is aggravated by diuretic therapy
    E some patients with chronic encephalopathy respond well to bromocriptine therapy

6   Gastric acid secretion
    A is principally under the control of the vagus nerve
    B is higher than normal in the majority of duodenal ulcer patients
    C is suppressed by antral acidification
    D is related to the total number of oxyntic cells in the stomach
    E is effected by an ATP-dependent cation transfer mechanism

7   Recognized hepatic complications of Crohn's disease include
    A cholelithiasis
    B primary biliary cirrhosis
    C cholangiocarcinoma
    D hepatic steatosis
    E pericholangitis

8   The following predispose to gastro-oesophageal reflux
    A truncal vagotomy
    B cigarette smoking
    C treatment of achalasia of the cardia
    D pregnancy
    E pyloric stenosis

9   In patients with Addisonian pernicious anaemia
    A circulating serum gastrin levels are low
    B there is an increased incidence of autoimmune thyroid disease
    C intrinsic factor antibodies are present in gastric juice
    D the absorption of vitamin B_{12} is improved by immunosuppressive therapy
    E the prevalence of associated duodenal ulcer is 10%

5 A **False** in a dosage of 2 mg/kg, it reduces portal venous pressure
   B **False** there is an association between chronic active hepatitis and renal tubular acidosis and between congenital hepatic fibrosis and medullary sponge kidney
   C **False** gynaecomastia is thought to reflect the oestrogenic properties of most sex hormone metabolites
   D **True**   this is due to reduction in renal blood flow secondary to plasma volume depletion
   E **True**   although the response is unpredictable

6 A **False** gastrin and other gastrointestinal hormones play an important part in gastric secretory control
   B **False** two-thirds of patients with duodenal ulceration have acid outputs within the normal range
   C **True**   inhibits the release of gastrin
   D **True**
   E **True**   the site of action of the proton pump inhibitor omeprazole

7 A **True**   related to changes in the circulating bile acid pool, in patients with terminal ileum involvement
   B **False** secondary biliary cirrhosis may occur as a result of pericholangitis or gall stones
   C **True**   secondary to disturbances of the circulating bile acid pool
   D **True**   a reflection of malnutrition
   E **True**   the pathogenesis is ill understood

8 A **True**   denervation of the lower oesophageal sphincter (LOS)
   B **True**   nicotine reduces the LOS pressure
   C **True**   both pneumatic dilatation and cardiomyotomy may result in reflux
   D **True**   increased intra-abdominal pressure and hormonal effects on LOS pressure
   E **True**   due to decreased gastric emptying

9 A **False** achlorhydria results in increased gastrin release
   B **True**
   C **True**   binding and blocking antibodies in gastric secretions, reduce vitamin B_{12} absorption
   D **True**   it suppresses the autoimmune process
   E **False** no acid, no ulcer

10   In cystic fibrosis
  A   the incidence is 1 in 20 000 live births
  B   respiratory symptoms develop during the first year of life in the majority of patients
  C   repeated attacks of intestinal obstruction are a recognized complication in adults
  D   male infertility is characteristic
  E   survival beyond the age of 20 is rare

11   Recognized associations of ulcerative colitis include
  A   the presence of circulating immune complexes
  B   an increased mortality in the first attack in patients over the age of 60
  C   an increased risk of large-bowel carcinoma
  D   reduction of the progression of associated ankylosing spondylitis following panproctocolectomy
  E   primary sclerosing cholangitis

12   Typical gastrointestinal manifestations of systemic sclerosis include
  A   oesophageal stricture
  B   primary biliary cirrhosis
  C   abnormal exocrine pancreatic function tests
  D   diverticulae of the large bowel
  E   small-bowel visceral myopathy

13   Anal continence is
  A   principally under voluntary control
  B   impaired in faecal impaction of the rectum
  C   dependent on the integrity of the internal anal sphincter
  D   affected by stool consistency
  E   impaired in paraplegic patients with a lesion at mid-thoracic level

14   Gastrointestinal hormones mediate the following actions
  A   gastrin increases gastric motor activity
  B   gastric inhibitory polypeptide inhibits insulin secretion
  C   pancreatic polypeptide stimulates pancreatic bicarbonate secretion
  D   enteroglucagon decreases small-bowel transit
  E   secretin maintains mucosal growth

10	A	**False**	the incidence is about 1 in 2000 live births
	B	**True**	
	C	**True**	'adult meconium ileus' due to luminal obstruction by inspissated secretions
	D	**True**	caused by defective cilial function of spermatozoa
	E	**False**	60% of patients now survive beyond the age of 20. Lung transplantation can have a useful role

11	A	**True**	these complexes may be related to the associated arthritis and to pyoderma gangrenosum
	B	**True**	the mortality in these patients is approximately 15%
	C	**True**	the highest risk is in those patients who have had a pancolitis for over 10 years
	D	**False**	the activity of one is independent of the activity of the other
	E	**True**	

12	A	**True**	this is due to destruction of the smooth muscle of the lower oesophageal sphincter and disordered oesophageal peristalsis
	B	**True**	especially if associated with CREST syndrome
	C	**True**	about one-third of patients have abnormal pancreatic function tests
	D	**True**	characteristically these are wide-mouthed pseudo-diverticula on the anti-mesenteric border in the transverse and descending colon
	E	**True**	associated with significant hypomotility, malabsorption and steatorrhoea

13	A	**False**	the internal sphincter is under autonomic control while the external sphincter is under voluntary control
	B	**True**	spurious diarrhoea and overflow incontinence may occur as a result of faecal impaction
	C	**True**	
	D	**True**	fluid stools may be associated with incontinence
	E	**False**	in the absence of faecal impaction, continence is dependent on a spinal reflex at sacral level

14	A	**True**	it also stimulates acid secretion and maintains mucosal growth
	B	**False**	it stimulates insulin secretion
	C	**False**	it inhibits pancreatic secretion and gall bladder contractility
	D	**True**	and maintains mucosal growth
	E	**False**	secretin stimulates pancreatic bicarbonate secretion

15   Urinobilinogen excretion is reduced or absent in the urine in jaundice due to
A   autoimmune haemolytic anaemia
B   Crigler–Najjar syndrome
C   carcinoma of the head of the pancreas
D   hepatic cirrhosis
E   chlorpromazine

16   A woman of 45 with a long history of alcohol abuse and depression was commenced on chlorpromazine therapy. One month later the serum bilirubin was 340 μmol/l, alanine aminotransferase 250 U/l and alkaline phosphatase 300 U/l. The urine contained bilirubin and an excess of urobilinogen. These findings suggest a diagnosis of
A   alcoholic hepatitis
B   chlorpromazine induced jaundice
C   carcinoma of the common bile duct
D   haemolytic anaemia
E   hepatocellular carcinoma

17   In chronic pancreatitis
A   cholelithiasis is the commonest aetiological factor
B   the majority of patients have an abnormal glucose tolerance test 10 years or more after onset
C   small-bowel biopsy is often abnormal
D   the diagnosis is best confirmed by radio-isotope scanning of the pancreas
E   severe malabsorption only develops when enzyme secretion is reduced by over 90%

18   In functional hepatorenal failure (hepatorenal syndrome)
A   urinary sodium excretion increases
B   plasma renin activity is elevated
C   endotoxinaemia is an important contributory factor
D   renal cortical necrosis is a recognized complication
E   treatment with high-dose frusemide is indicated

19   A 25-year-old man presents with a 2-week history of diarrhoea with blood and mucus. He had spent 3 years in Nigeria and recently returned to the UK. On examination he is ill, temperature 38.5°C, clinically anaemic and has generalized abdominal tenderness
A   treatment with intravenous hydrocortisone should be started immediately
B   the presence of discrete rectal ulcers at sigmoidoscopy suggests a diagnosis of ulcerative colitis
C   emergency panproctocolectomy is indicated
D   polyarthritis of the lower limbs suggests the diagnosis of inflammatory bowel disease
E   plain X-rays of the abdomen are mandatory

15 A **False** increased due to conjugated bilirubin metabolism
    B **True** absence of glucuronyl transferase
    C **True** ⎫
    D **True** ⎬ obstruction to bilirubin excretion
    E **True** ⎭

16 A **True** the mixed hepatic and obstructive features of the
                 liver function tests are typical
    B **False** ⎫ the excess of urobilinogen in the urine and the marked
                 increase in the ALT levels make these diagnoses
    C **False** ⎭ unlikely
    D **False** the biochemical profile suggests a liver disorder
    E **False** possible but unlikely

17 A **False** alcohol abuse is the predominant factor
    B **True** about two-thirds have a diabetic oral glucose
                 tolerance test
    C **False**
    D **False** CT and ultrasound scanning of the pancreas are
                 much better
    E **True**

18 A **False** the urinary sodium excretion is less than 20 mmol/l
    B **True** the mechanism is unclear
    C **True**
    D **False** acute tubular necrosis may supervene
    E **False** this may precipitate acute tubular necrosis

19 A **False** amoebic colitis is the diagnosis until proved
                 otherwise
    B **False** such ulcers suggest either Crohn's, Behçet's, or
                 amoebic colitis
    C **False**
    D **True** a mono-arthritis raises the possibility of septic
                 arthritis
    E **True** to exclude both toxic dilatation of the colon and
                 perforation

20   In patients with the short bowel syndrome the following are expected findings
- A   gastric hypersecretion
- B   an increased incidence of gallstones
- C   diarrhoea which responds to treatment with cholestyramine
- D   vitamin B_{12} deficiency
- E   an increased incidence of renal stones

21   The incidence of squamous carcinoma of the oesophagus is increased in
- A   coeliac disease
- B   South Africans
- C   achalasia of the cardia
- D   Barrett's oesophagus
- E   tylosis palmaris et plantaris

22   In bilirubin metabolism
- A   85% of bilirubin is derived from haemoglobin degradation
- B   hepatic uptake of bilirubin is mediated by specific binding proteins
- C   conjugated bilirubin is well absorbed from the terminal ileum
- D   unconjugated bilirubin is excreted by the kidneys
- E   conjugation occurs in the endoplasmic reticulum of hepatocytes

23   In simple diverticulosis of the colon
- A   a high-fibre diet accelerates colonic transit time
- B   the presence of symptoms suggests either an alternative or additional diagnosis
- C   intermittent rectal bleeding is an expected finding
- D   the condition exists in 50% of the UK population over the age of 60
- E   there is an increased incidence in black Africans

24   In Wilson's disease
- A   alpha-1-antitrypsin levels are increased
- B   plasma caeruloplasmin levels are increased
- C   corneal copper deposits are present in the majority of patients
- D   the presence of excess amounts of copper in the liver is diagnostic
- E   treatment with trientine is reserved for patients with established hepatic cirrhosis

20 A **True** due to loss of inhibition of gastric acid secretion by small intestinal hormones

B **True** due to depletion of the bile salt pool, secretion of lithogenic bile is increased

C **True** diarrhoea is exacerbated by unabsorbed bile salts in the colon

D **True** absorption is also impaired by the bacterial colonization of the remaining small bowel

E **True** secondary to increased colonic oxalate absorption and hyperoxaluria

21 A **True** increased incidence of all upper gastrointestinal tract carcinomas as well as small bowel lymphoma

B **True** the incidence is increased particularly in black Africans but also in white South Africans

C **True** increased risk of 5- to 10-fold

D **False** associated with an increased incidence of adenocarcinoma

E **True** rare disorder of keratinization

22 A **True** the rest derives from myoglobin and cytochromes

B **True** there are two (Y and Z) called ligandins

C **False** it is a polar molecule, hydrolysed by colonic bacteria and absorbed and excreted as urinobilinogen

D **False** conjugated bilirubin is excreted by the kidney

E **True** a microsomal process

23 A **True**

B **True** usually completely asymptomatic if uncomplicated

C **False** the possibility of coexisting colonic carcinoma or angiodysplasia must always be considered

D **True** the statistic applies to Western populations

E **False** in rural Africans who live on a high-residue diet the condition is almost unknown

24 A **False** it is an alpha-1-globulin, synthesized in the liver and levels are low or normal in chronic liver disease

B **False** they are low and considered the basic metabolic defect

C **True** copper deposits in Descemet's membrane produce the Kayser–Fleischer rings

D **False** increased amounts of copper in the liver also occur in primary and secondary biliary cirrhosis

E **False** treatment should be started as soon as the diagnosis is made, to prevent cirrhosis. Trientine is reserved for patients intolerant of penicillamine

25   **A man of 60 presents with a 6-month history of pale offensive bowel motions and weight loss of 8 kg. The following findings are compatible with the history**
    A   normal small-bowel barium enema
    B   jejunal biopsy showing sub-total villous atrophy
    C   faecal fat excretion 72 mmol/day
    D   abnormal ^{14}C glycocholate breath test
    E   improvement with metronidazole therapy

26   **Typical features of pellagra include**
    A   photosensitive dermatitis
    B   night blindness
    C   watery diarrhoea
    D   bleeding gums
    E   dependent oedema

27   **In Whipple's disease**
    A   middle-aged women are most frequently affected
    B   Gram-negative cocci are the causative organisms
    C   PAS-staining granules are present in the macrophages throughout the body
    D   ophthalmoplegia, polyarthritis and pulmonary manifestations are recognized complications
    E   treatment with broad-spectrum antibiotics should be continued for 12 months

28   **The following features are characteristic of fulminant hepatic failure**
    A   asterixis
    B   hypoglycaemia
    C   variceal bleeding
    D   hyperventilation
    E   prolongation of prothrombin time

29   **Recognized gastrointestinal associations of hyperparathyroidism include**
    A   gall stones
    B   constipation
    C   acute pancreatitis
    D   duodenal ulceration attributable to hypergastrinaemia
    E   diarrhoea attributable to hypercalcitoninaemia

25 A **True** malabsorption secondary to chronic pancreatic disease
   B **True** coeliac disease can present with features suggesting severe malabsorption
   C **True**
   D **True** bacterial colonization of the small bowel
   E **True** giardiasis can produce malabsorption, as may bacterial overgrowth

26 A **True** the dermatitis on the neck above the shirt line is known as Casal's necklace
   B **False** a feature of vitamin A deficiency
   C **True** due to the effect of niacin deficiency on the bowel epithelium
   D **False** a feature of scurvy
   E **False** a feature of beri-beri (thiamine deficiency)

27 A **False** mainly middle-aged men
   B **False** Gram-positive rod-shaped bacilli
   C **True**
   D **True**
   E **True** recommended therapy includes penicillin and streptomycin or tetracycline for 6–12 months

28 A **True** a flapping tremor is seen until coma supervenes
   B **True** may be severe, contributes to coma and reflects impaired hepatic gluconeogenesis
   C **False** portal hypertension is rare; gastrointestinal bleeding is usually from acute gastric erosions
   D **True** due to cerebral oedema
   E **True**

29 A **False** increased incidence of renal stones only
   B **True** an effect of hypercalcaemia on intestinal motility
   C **True** due to ectopic calcification
   D **True** association with gastrinoma and MEN I
   E **True** association with medullary carcinoma of thyroid gland (MEN II)

30   In acute upper gastrointestinal haemorrhage
- A   intravenous ranitidine reduces the incidence of rebleeding within 10 days of the initial bleed
- B   the mortality rate increases with the age of the patient
- C   the presence of stigmata of chronic liver disease indicates that the likeliest cause of bleeding is oesophageal varices
- D   somatostatin infusion can help to control bleeding
- E   5–10% of patients bleed from Mallory–Weiss oesophageal tears

31   In viral hepatitis
- A   hepatitis A is usually transmitted by infected blood products
- B   there is an increased incidence of hepatitis C in patients with haemophilia
- C   50% of adults infected with hepatitis B become chronic carriers
- D   there is an increased incidence of hepatocellular carcinoma in chronic HBsAg carriers
- E   hepatitis A infections are a recognized sequel of shellfish ingestion

32   In chronic alcoholics
- A   the prevalence of liver disease is 80%
- B   sensitivity to sedative drugs is decreased
- C   changes of hepatitis on liver histology are associated with a better prognosis than changes of steatosis
- D   the liver damage is principally due to associated dietary deficiencies
- E   the pattern of drinking is important in determining the development of liver disease

33   Abnormalities of liver function tests are a recognized feature of
- A   rifampicin therapy
- B   polymyalgia rheumatica
- C   the second trimester of pregnancy
- D   thyrotoxicosis
- E   poorly controlled diabetes mellitus

30 A **False**
   B **True**   the mortality is lowest in patients under 40 and is highest in patients aged 70 years or over
   C **False** patients with chronic liver disease bleed from other lesions even if they are known to have varices
   D **True**
   E **True**

31 A **False** ⎤ hepatitis B and hepatitis C are commonly
   B **True** ⎦ transmitted by infected blood products
   C **False** only about 5% of infected adults become chronic carriers
   D **True**   this is one of the commonest carcinomas in areas where hepatitis B is endemic
   E **True**   shellfish filter the virus from polluted waters

32 A **False** approximately half of chronic alcoholics in psychiatric hospitals have no evidence of liver disease
   B **True**   hepatic microsomal enzyme induction
   C **False** fatty liver is potentially reversible; severe alcoholic hepatitis carries a poor prognosis
   D **False** the liver damage is principally related to the amount of alcohol consumed
   E **True**   'binge' drinkers seem to have less severe liver disease than continuous drinkers

33 A **True**   elevated transaminase levels are common
   B **True**   one-third of patients have an elevated alkaline phosphatase level
   C **False** a rise in alkaline phosphatase level may occur in the third trimester
   D **True**   minor abnormalities are common
   E **True**   acute fatty liver returns to normal when the diabetes is better controlled

34 Elevation of the serum amylase is a recognized finding in
A   mumps
B   acute renal failure
C   hypothermia
D   diabetic ketoacidosis
E   alcoholic hepatitis

35 Needle biopsy of the liver
A   should be avoided in suspected hydatid disease
B   is the investigation of choice in extrahepatic obstructive jaundice
C   has a mortality rate of 1%
D   is a useful investigation in adult Gaucher's disease
E   should be avoided if metastatic liver disease is suspected

36 Acute pancreatitis is
A   associated with azathioprine therapy
B   a recognized cause of tetany
C   invariably associated with hyperamylasaemia
D   best treated with opiate analgesics and fluid replacement
E   associated with a worse prognosis in elderly patients

37 Typical features of familial Mediterranean fever include
A   autosomal dominant inheritance
B   presentation with abdominal pain and arthralgias
C   erysipelas-like erythema of lower limbs
D   beneficial response to prednisolone
E   affects Caucasians more often than Blacks

38 Carcinoid syndrome
A   occurs in the majority of patients with carcinoid tumours
B   is an expected finding in colorectal carcinoids with liver metastases
C   is associated with a pellagra-like state
D   is improved by hepatic artery ligation
E   has a survival of less than 2 years from diagnosis

34 A **True** salivary amylase is a different isoenzyme from pancreatic amylase
   B **True** amylase is excreted by the kidney
   C **True** painless
   D **True** ketone bodies interfere with the laboratory estimation of amylase
   E **True** transient hyperamylasaemia may occur in acute alcoholic intoxication and alcohol-associated acute pancreatitis

35 A **True** there is a risk of anaphylactic shock and dissemination of infection
   B **False**
   C **False** the mortality rate with a Menghini needle is approximately 0.02%
   D **True** typical Gaucher's cells seen
   E **False** it can be used in combination with ultrasound or even laparoscopy to biopsy suspicious areas

36 A **True** idiosyncratic response
   B **True** if fat necrosis is severe
   C **False**
   D **True** the relief of pain is the first priority despite any increase in intrabiliary pressure
   E **True**

37 A **False** autosomal recessive
   B **True** it is a polyserositis which may affect any serosal surface
   C **True** about 25%
   D **False** the treatment of choice is colchicine
   E **True** affects Mediterraneans, including Greeks, Turks and Italians

38 A **False** the syndrome occurs in about 5% of patients with carcinoid tumours
   B **False** colorectal carcinoid tumours are functionally different from other carcinoids and do not produce 5HT
   C **True** increased tryptophan metabolism results in reduced niacin synthesis
   D **True** the metastases in the liver are dependent on the hepatic artery for their blood supply
   E **False** most patients survive between 5 and 10 years and survival for as long as 20 years has been recorded

39   In the diagnosis of rapidly increasing jaundice
   A   liver function values reliably distinguish obstructive from hepatocellular causes
   B   ultrasound examination of the liver is the investigation of choice
   C   the absence of bilirubinuria suggests hepatitis
   D   percutaneous transhepatic cholangiography is unlikely to be successful in the absence of dilated ducts on ultrasound examination
   E   endoscopic retrograde cholangiography should be avoided in the elderly

40   In haemochromatosis
   A   males are more severely affected
   B   there is an increased frequency of HLA B8
   C   splenomegaly is a characteristic finding
   D   young patients may present with congestive cardiomyopathy
   E   liver transplantation is the treatment of choice

39 A **False** the differentiation can be difficult
   B **True** the presence of dilated intrahepatic ducts on
           ultrasound suggests an obstructive cause
   C **False** acute haemolysis
   D **False** normal calibre intrahepatic ducts can be delineated
   E **False** ERCP is a better option than surgery in the elderly

40 A **True** menstrual loss in women may retard the
           accumulation of iron stores
   B **False** increased HLA A3
   C **False** unlike hepatomegaly, splenomegaly is uncommon
   D **True**
   E **False** regular venesection to prevent iron accumulation is
           more appropriate

Haematology

1   Recognized findings in the peripheral blood in severe folic acid deficiency include
   A   microcytosis
   B   thrombocytopenia
   C   anisocytosis
   D   megaloblastosis
   E   subnormal serum vitamin B_{12} concentration

2   Microangiopathic haemolytic anaemia is a recognized finding in
   A   disseminated intravascular coagulation
   B   thrombotic thrombocytopenic purpura
   C   the haemolytic uraemic syndrome
   D   disseminated carcinoma
   E   malignant hypertension

3   Characteristic complications of severe sickle-cell anaemia include
   A   infective dactylitis
   B   aseptic necrosis of the femoral heads
   C   chronic leg ulcers
   D   pulmonary fibrosis
   E   liver cell necrosis

4   Causes of megaloblastic anaemia include
   A   phenytoin therapy
   B   myxoedema
   C   ibuprofen therapy
   D   hereditary orotic aciduria
   E   infestation with *Diphyllobothrium latum*

5   In polycythaemia rubra vera
   A   arterial oxygen saturation is reduced
   B   the serum uric acid is often elevated
   C   the neutrophil alkaline phosphatase score is characteristically low
   D   there is usually a leucocytosis and thrombocytosis
   E   the plasma volume is increased

1	A	**False**	anaemia with marked oval macrocytosis, anisocytosis and poikilocytosis
	B	**True**	thrombocytopenia is usually mild and benign
	C	**True**	
	D	**True**	occasionally megaloblasts are seen in the peripheral blood
	E	**True**	the serum B_{12} is subnormal in 40% of cases due to the interrelated metabolism of B_{12} and folate

2	A	**True**	characterized by red cell fragmentation, fibrin deposition in the small vessels and DIC
	B	**True**	platelet aggregates surrounded by fibrin cause arteriolar occlusions
	C	**True**	due to endothelial changes in glomerular capillaries and renal arterioles
	D	**True**	
	E	**True**	fibrinoid necrosis

3	A	**True**	non-infective dactylitis due to microinfarction also occurs
	B	**True**	bone infarction
	C	**True**	usually on the medial surface of the lower tibia
	D	**True**	associated with pulmonary hypertension
	E	**True**	more rarely fulminant hepatic failure

4	A	**True**	induction of folate metabolism
	B	**False**	macrocytosis but not anaemia unless associated with vitamin B_{12} deficiency
	C	**False**	
	D	**True**	an inherited disorder of pyrimidine metabolism unresponsive to folate or vitamin B_{12}
	E	**True**	a fish tapeworm of Finland, causing malabsorption of vitamin B_{12}

5	A	**False**	normal PO_2 in PRV in contrast to the low PO_2 in patients with chronic pulmonary or cardiac disease
	B	**True**	increased purine metabolism
	C	**False**	usually elevated
	D	**True**	PRV is associated with a hyperplastic marrow
	E	**False**	the plasma volume is usually normal or reduced

6   Leukaemoid blood reactions are associated with
  A   tuberculosis
  B   disseminated malignancy
  C   severe burns
  D   massive haemorrhage
  E   neutrophilia with the presence of the Philadelphia chromosome

7   In the red blood cells
  A   Heinz bodies indicate denatured haemoglobin
  B   Howell–Jolly bodies are remnants of nuclear material
  C   poikilocytosis describes an alteration in the size of blood cells
  D   the mean corpuscular haemoglobin concentration is reduced in hereditary spherocytosis
  E   basophilic stippling is a characteristic finding in lead poisoning

8   Typical findings in haemolytic anaemia include
  A   elevation of the serum haptoglobin
  B   haemosiderin in the urine
  C   hyperbilirubinaemia of the unconjugated type
  D   erythroid hypoplasia of the marrow
  E   increased urinary urobilinogen

9   A hypochromic microcytic blood film would be an expected finding in
  A   beta-thalassaemia
  B   primary (hereditary) sideroblastic anaemia
  C   lead poisoning
  D   chronic infection
  E   paroxysmal nocturnal haemoglobinuria

10   The erythrocyte sedimentation rate (ESR) is
  A   elevated in sickle-cell anaemia
  B   depressed in Waldenstrom's macroglobulinaemia
  C   elevated in polycythaemia
  D   useful in monitoring the progress of temporal arteritis
  E   invariably elevated in myeloma

6 A **True** leukaemoid reactions without the typical marrow changes of leukaemia occur in tuberculosis, whooping cough, diphtheria, infectious mononucleosis, severe burns, eclampsia, neoplastic bone marrow involvement and severe haemorrhage or haemolysis

B **True**

C **True**

D **True**

E **False** Ph chromosome is not specific for CML but never occurs in non-neoplastic marrow dyscrasias

7 A **True** Heinz bodies are caused by oxidant drugs and are also associated with the unstable haemoglobins and thalassaemias

B **True** particularly after splenectomy

C **False** poikilocytosis is an alteration in the shape of red blood cells

D **False** spherocytes have a mean corpuscular haemoglobin concentration which is increased

E **True**

8 A **False** the serum haptoglobin falls as the plasma haemoglobin rises

B **True** haemoglobin passed through the glomeruli is metabolized to haemosiderin in renal tubules

C **True**

D **False** the marrow is typically hyperplastic

E **True** in acholuric jaundice, bilirubin bound to albumin cannot pass the renal glomeruli; excess conjugated bilirubin is metabolized to urobilinogen

9 A **True** reduced synthesis of β globin chains resulting in red blood cells deficient in haemoglobin

B **True** the hereditary form of sideroblastic anaemia is microcytic and hypochromic; the idiopathic form is normocytic or macrocytic

C **True** haem synthesis is depressed

D **False** usually normocytic and normochromic

E **False** macrocytic blood picture, although hypochromia and microcytosis occasionally occur

10 A **False** the ESR is low as sickle cells are unable to form rouleaux

B **False** the ESR is elevated in disorders of plasma proteins, e.g. myeloma or macroglobulinaemia

C **False** the ESR is usually low

D **True**

E **False**

11   Recognized features of chronic lymphocytic leukaemia include
   A   defective antibody production
   B   Coombs' positive haemolytic anaemia
   C   improved survival of asymptomatic patients given
         chemotherapy
   D   ampicillin hypersensitivity
   E   leukaemic infiltrations of pleura and pericardium

12   An increased incidence of leukaemia is associated with
   A   Down's syndrome
   B   fetal irradiation
   C   Epstein–Barr virus infection
   D   treatment for Hodgkin's disease
   E   extreme old age

13   Hodgkin's disease
   A   is commoner in women than men
   B   most often involves the cervical lymph nodes
   C   is confirmed histologically by the presence of
         Reed–Sternberg cells
   D   is associated with pruritus
   E   is best treated by radiotherapy if the marrow is involved

14   An increased red cell mass is seen in
   A   cerebellar haemangioblastoma
   B   Gaisbock's syndrome
   C   chronic mountain sickness
   D   congenital heart disease
   E   uterine fibroids

15   Typical findings in myelofibrosis include
   A   leucoerythroblastic peripheral blood picture
   B   splenomegaly
   C   thrombocytopenia
   D   peripheral blood poikilocytosis
   E   a low leucocyte alkaline phosphatase score

11 A **True** marked tendency to infection
  B **True** approximately 10%
  C **False** specific chemotherapy in CLL does not prolong survival
  D **True** maculopapular rash is characteristic
  E **True**

12 A **True**
  B **True** especially CML
  C **False** Burkitt's lymphoma
  D **True** especially AML
  E **False**

13 A **False** the male/female sex ratio ranges from 1.4 to 1.9:1
  B **True**
  C **True**
  D **True** can be a presenting feature
  E **False** stage 4 disease indicates diffuse or disseminated involvement of one or more extralymphatic organ or tissue with or without associated lymph node involvement and should be treated by chemotherapy

14 A **True** erythropoietic activity in the cystic tumour
  B **False** relative polycythaemia; the red cell mass is normal and the plasma volume is reduced
  C **True** increased plasma erythropoietin levels
  D **True** response to low PaO_2
  E **True** erythropoietic activity in fibroids

15 A **True** nucleated red blood cells and myelocytes in the peripheral blood
  B **True** myelofibrosis and chronic myeloid leukaemia often produce massive splenomegaly
  C **False** the platelet count is usually high
  D **True**
  E **False** an elevated or normal leucocyte alkaline phosphatase and absence of the Philadelphia chromosome help to distinguish myelofibrosis from chronic myeloid leukaemia

16   Recognized features of multiple myeloma include
A   bone pain
B   renal amyloidosis
C   a poor prognosis in anaemic patients
D   a monoclonal gammopathy with an immune paresis
E   peak incidence in the fourth decade

17   A mean corpuscular volume (MCV) of greater than 100 femtolitres is a recognized feature of
A   iron-deficiency anaemia
B   chronic liver disease
C   pure red cell aplasia
D   reticulocytosis
E   thyroxine deficiency

18   Splenectomy is helpful in the management of
A   acquired autoimmune haemolytic anaemia
B   hereditary spherocytosis
C   sickle-cell anaemia
D   chronic idiopathic thrombocytopenic purpura
E   pyruvate kinase deficiency

19   Hyposplenism is associated with
A   target cells
B   systemic lupus erythematosus
C   Howell–Jolly bodies
D   gluten enteropathy
E   Fanconi's anaemia

20   Recognized features of untreated Addisonian pernicious anaemia include
A   gastric acid secretion in response to pentagastrin stimulation
B   weight loss
C   Schilling test invariably corrects with intrinsic factor
D   megaloblastic anaemia
E   pancytopenia

16 A **True**   a major presenting symptom together with anaemia, uraemia and infection
  B **True**   amyloidosis occurs in about 10%
  C **True**
  D **True**   the monoclonal gammopathy is associated with a reduction in the other immunoglobulins
  E **False**   the incidence peaks during the seventh decade

---

17 A **False**   microcytosis
  B **True**   particularly in association with alcoholism
  C **True**
  D **True**
  E **True**

---

18 A **True**   of value when steroid therapy has failed
  B **True**   the treatment of choice and prolongs red cell survival
  C **False**   rarely in children with hypersplenism
  D **True**   if steroid therapy has failed or unacceptably high doses are required
  E **True**   successful in some cases

---

19 A **True**   post-splenectomy there is usually an increase in reticulocytes, and Howell–Jolly bodies and target cells are present
  B **False**   splenomegaly occurs in about 10% and may be associated with a haemolytic anaemia
  C **True**
  D **True**
  E **True**   Fanconi's anaemia is a congenital aplastic anaemia with skeletal abnormalities and skin pigmentation

---

20 A **False**   pentagastrin-resistant achlorhydria
  B **True**   weight loss is common
  C **False**   small-bowel mucosal changes may take 6–9 months to revert to normal
  D **True**
  E **True**   megaloblastosis often affects other bone marrow precursor cells resulting in a pancytopenia

21   Cerebral infarctions are recognized sequelae of
A   sickle-cell disease
B   thalassaemia minor
C   myelomatosis
D   paroxysmal nocturnal haemoglobinuria
E   thrombotic thrombocytopenic purpura

22   Characteristic laboratory features of disseminated intravascular coagulation include
A   normal thrombin time
B   reduced plasma fibrinogen
C   prolonged prothrombin time
D   thrombocytopenia
E   normal partial thromboplastin time

23   Expected findings in untreated chronic myeloid leukaemia include
A   increased platelet count
B   increased serum vitamin B_{12}
C   increased blood urea
D   monoclonal gammopathy
E   raised neutrophil alkaline phosphatase score

24   Recognized associations with pernicious anaemia include
A   immunodeficiency states
B   diabetes mellitus
C   gastric carcinoma
D   vitiligo
E   atrophic hypothyroidism

25   In paroxysmal nocturnal haemoglobinuria
A   the red cells are hypersensitive to changes in pH
B   leucocytosis is common
C   urinary haemosiderin is elevated
D   the red cells are sensitive to complement-mediated haemolysis
E   the disorder is associated with a cold antibody

26   The bleeding time is characteristically prolonged in
A   haemophilia
B   warfarin therapy
C   Von Willebrand's disease
D   thrombocytopenia
E   factor X deficiency

21 A **True**   sickle cells sludge within the vasculature
   B **False**   usually asymptomatic
   C **True**   hyperviscosity syndrome
   D **True**   venous thromboses are common in PNH
   E **True**   often a presenting feature

22 A **False**   disseminated intravascular coagulation (DIC) is
                 associated with a reduced fibrinogen level and a
                 prolonged thrombin time and PTT
   B **True**
   C **True**
   D **True**
   E **False**

23 A **True**   in approximately 50%
   B **True**   increased levels of transcobalamin
   C **False**   <u>urate</u> may be elevated however
   D **False**
   E **False**   neutrophil alkaline phosphatase score is reduced or
                 absent in 90%

24 A **True**   PA has occasionally been associated with an adult
                 onset hypogammaglobulinaemia, diabetes mellitus
                 and Addison's disease
   B **True**
   C **True**   patients with PA have a 4-fold increase in gastric
                 carcinoma
   D **True**
   E **True**

25 A **True**   PNH cells are lysed in acidified human serum
   B **False**   granulocytes like red blood cells in PNH are sensitive
                 to complement lysis and leucopenia is common
   C **True**   intravascular haemolysis
   D **True**
   E **False**   abnormal RBC clones

26 A **False**   bleeding time is a measure of platelet count, platelet
                 function and vascular integrity
   B **False**   inhibits vitamin K and the formation of factors II, VII,
                 IX and X
   C **True**   associated with platelet function defect
   D **True**
   E **False**   the bleeding time is usually normal

27   **The following features suggest Von Willebrand's disease**
   A   a prolonged bleeding time
   B   spontaneous venous thromboses
   C   reduced ristocetin-induced platelet aggregation
   D   a normal factor VIIIvWFAg
   E   an autosomal dominant mode of inheritance

28   **The prothrombin time is increased in**
   A   warfarin therapy
   B   Christmas disease
   C   haemophilia
   D   liver failure
   E   heparin therapy

29   **Recognized findings in haemophilia include**
   A   normal prothrombin time
   B   normal platelet count
   C   prolonged bleeding time
   D   normal partial thromboplastin time
   E   prolonged euglobulin clot lysis time

30   **Disseminated intravascular coagulation is a characteristic complication of**
   A   antepartum haemorrhage
   B   meningococcal septicaemia
   C   metastatic prostatic carcinoma
   D   chronic myeloid leukaemia
   E   acute promyelocytic leukaemia

31   **In haemophilia A**
   A   the prothrombin time is prolonged
   B   haemarthrosis is rare
   C   Kaposi's sarcoma is rare in HIV-positive patients
   D   male offspring of known carriers are detected by fetal blood factor VIII levels
   E   freeze-dried factor VIII concentrate is given four times daily for 2 days before major elective surgery

27   A   **True**   Von Willebrand's disease is associated with a deficiency of plasma factor VIII procoagulant required for the adhesion of platelets to damaged vessels

     B   **False**   skin and mucus membrane <u>bleeding</u> occurs

     C   **True**   platelets suspended in Von Willebrand's plasma fail to aggregate with ristocetin

     D   **False**   reduced

     E   **True**   usually autosomal dominant unlike haemophilia

---

28   A   **True**   the prothrombin time measures the <u>extrinsic factors</u> in coagulation. Warfarin is an inhibitor of vitamin K-dependent factors <u>II, VII, IX and X,</u> synthesized in the liver

     B   **False**   a hereditary defect in the clotting activity of factor IX

     C   **False**   factor VIII is part of the <u>intrinsic</u> clotting system

     D   **True**

     E   **True**   heparin acts with antithrombin III and inhibits factors XIIa, XIa, IXa and Xa, thrombin and plasmin resulting in a prolonged thrombin time and partial thromboplastin time

---

29   A   **True**

     B   **True**

     C   **False**   clotting time (in vitro) not the bleeding time (in vivo) is prolonged

     D   **False**   the partial thromboplastin time measures the intrinsic system and is typically prolonged in haemophilia

     E   **False**   the euglobulin clot lysis time measures the activation of plasminogen activators

---

30   A   **True**   (DIC) is associated with antepartum haemorrhage, abruptio placenta, amniotic fluid embolism and eclampsia; the placenta is rich in thromboplastins

     B   **True**   many septicaemias can provoke DIC

     C   **True**   tumours contain thromboplastins

     D   **False**

     E   **True**   promyelocyte blast cell granules also contain thromboplastins

---

31   A   **False**   the activated partial thromboplastin time (APTT) is prolonged

     B   **False**

     C   **True**   the natural history of HIV infection in haemophilia is different

     D   **True**

     E   **False**   factor VIII half-life is 12 hours so twice daily is usually enough. Trough levels of factor VIIIc should be above 60% before major surgery

32 In idiopathic acquired hypoplastic anaemia
   A oxymethalone therapy improves the long-term prognosis
   B benign thymoma is a recognized cause
   C repeated red cell transfusions increase risk of bone marrow graft rejection
   D following glandular fever, spontaneous recovery is usual
   E splenomegaly is a typical feature

33 In acute lymphoblastic leukaemia (ALL)
   A the presence of the Philadelphia chromosome augurs a good prognosis
   B B cell ALL is the commonest form in adults
   C induction chemotherapy including L-asparaginase results in remission in a high percentage of patients
   D intrathecal methotrexate treatment is preferred to cranio-spinal irradiation to consolidate remission
   E testicular irradiation in boys has little impact on survival

34 In allogeneic bone marrow transplantation
   A low-grade graft-versus-host disease (GVHD) is advantageous to survival
   B younger patients have a poorer prognosis
   C granulocyte function does not return to normal for several years
   D early infection with cytomegalovirus is best treated with gancyclovir
   E acute GVHD presents with exfoliative dermatitis

35 In chronic myeloid leukaemia
   A promyelocytes are seen on the blood film
   B priapism is a recognized presenting feature
   C lymphadenopathy is a characteristic feature
   D DNA analysis demonstrates the chimeric Abelson-BCR gene
   E alpha interferon treatment induces remission

36 Target cells in the blood film are a feature of
   A splenectomy
   B cryptogenic cirrhosis
   C sickle-cell anaemia
   D thalassaemia minor
   E acquired haemolytic anaemia

32 A **False** proof of efficacy is lacking. Bone marrow
                  transplantation early in severe cases is advised
    B **True**   particularly if pure red cell aplasia
    C **True**   although usually unavoidable
    D **True**
    E **False**

33 A **False** occurs in 20% of adult ALL and indicates a poor
                  prognosis
    B **False** this is a rare form of ALL in both children and adults
    C **True**   in over 85% adults
    D **False** both should be given
    E **True**   and causes infertility and hypogonadism

34 A **True**   chronic GVHD is useful in preventing disease relapse
                  in some patients
    B **False** older patients do worse after BMT
    C **False** granulocyte function is regained by 3–4 weeks and
                  lymphocyte function by 3 years
    D **False** the risk of marrow toxicity is too great
    E **True**   cholestasis, hepatitis and diarrhoea also occur

35 A **True**   it is a proliferative rather than a maturation phase
                  disorder
    B **True**   about 2% of males present with this
    C **False** this is rare and more common in chronic
                  lymphocytic leukaemia
    D **True**   Abelson oncogene from chromosome 9 and
                  breakpoint cluster region (BCR) from chromosome
                  22 is the Philadelphia chromosome
    E **False** used to maintain control after remission with
                  busulphan or hydroxyurea

36 A **True**   seen in impaired or absent spleen function
    B **True**
    C **True** }
    D **True** } a feature of most haemoglobinopathies
    E **False**

37   An elevated eosinophil count is seen in
A   eosinophilic fasciitis
B   rubella
C   Löffler's endocarditis
D   hypothyroidism
E   chronic lymphocytic leukaemia

38   Basophilic stippling of erythrocytes on the blood film is a feature of
A   autoimmune haemolytic anaemia
B   lead poisoning
C   splenic atrophy
D   glucose-6-phosphate dehydrogenase deficiency
E   abetalipoproteinaemia

39   Characteristic features of beta-thalassaemia minor include
A   aseptic femoral head necrosis
B   elevated levels of HbF
C   renal papillary infarction
D   hypochromic anaemia
E   splenomegaly

40   Typical features of non-Hodgkin's lymphoma in adults include
A   leukaemic transformation at presentation
B   extranodal disease at presentation in about one-third of patients
C   need for staging laparoscopy and splenectomy
D   hilar lymphadenopathy on chest X-ray
E   paraplegia due to extradural tumour

37   A   **True**
     B   **False**   usually parasitic or mycobacterial but not viral
     C   **True**   the hypereosinophilic syndrome
     D   **False**   this may raise <u>basophil</u> counts
     E   **False**

38   A   **True**   basophilic stippling indicates accelerated
                      erythropoiesis or defective haemoglobin synthesis
     B   **True**
     C   **False**
     D   **True**
     E   **False**

39   A   **False**   individuals with the thalassaemia trait (minor) are
                      usually fit and well, with mild anaemia
     B   **False**
     C   **False**
     D   **True**
     E   **False**

40   A   **False**   rare event
     B   **True**
     C   **False**   unnecessary; most already have extensive disease
                      and require chemotherapy
     D   **False**   unlike Hodgkin's lymphoma
     E   **True**

Infectious diseases

1 **Characteristic features of infection with *Legionella pneumophila* include**
  A incubation period of 2–10 days
  B profuse diarrhoea
  C microscopic haematuria
  D raised plasma sodium
  E relative peripheral blood lymphocytosis

2 **In the management of purulent meningitis**
  A all cases are notifiable
  B contacts of meningococcal meningitis should be treated
  C severely ill patients should receive 1 megaunit of benzyl penicillin intrathecally
  D chloramphenicol should be avoided because of the risk of aplastic anaemia
  E the organism must be identified before treatment is commenced

3 **Live attenuated vaccines used in immunization include**
  A measles
  B tetanus
  C rubella
  D typhoid
  E hepatitis B

4 **In kala-azar (visceral leishmaniasis)**
  A transmission is by the bite of an infected female sandfly
  B infection occurs exclusively in tropical climates
  C the illness is characteristically afebrile
  D the diagnosis is best confirmed by liver biopsy
  E the treatment of choice is sodium stibogluconate

5 **Recognized complications of infectious mononucleosis include**
  A splenic rupture
  B myocarditis
  C polyneuritis
  D meningitis
  E glomerulonephritis

1 A **True**
  B **True**   headache, myalgia, cough, confusion, abdominal
            pain, vomiting and profuse diarrhoea may all occur
  C **True**   a high ESR, raised white cell count with
            relative lymphopenia, reduced plasma sodium
  D **False** and serum albumin levels; proteinuria and
  E **False** microscopic haematuria are often present

2 A **True**
  B **True**   chemoprophylaxis with rifampicin is advised
  C **False** the use of intrathecal penicillin is dangerous and
            unnecessary
  D **False** chloramphenicol is useful for haemophilus
            meningitis and in those allergic to penicillin
  E **False** CSF should be obtained but treatment is not
            withheld pending results

3 A **True**
  B **False** inactivated toxoid
  C **True**
  D **False** ⎫
  E **False** ⎭ both are inactivated preparations

4 A **True**
  B **False** also occurs in South America, the Mediterranean
            Islands and Southern Europe
  C **False**
  D **False** bone marrow is the safest means of isolating the
            organism, spleen smears the most productive
  E **True**

5 A **True** ⎫ complications include: splenic rupture,
            myocarditis, pericarditis,
  B **True**   polyneuritis, cranial nerve palsies, meningitis,
            encephalitis, transverse myelitis, glomerulonephritis
  C **True**   and polyarthritis, interstitial nephritis and
            pneumonitis, pharyngeal
  D **True**   oedema and respiratory obstruction,
            haemolytic anaemia, agranulocytosis,
  E **True** ⎭ agammaglobulinaemia and thrombocytopenia

6   In rubella
A   human immunoglobulin provides an effective protection against infection in pregnancy
B   a short (2–3 day) illness is usual
C   polyarthritis is the commonest complication in adults
D   successful immunisation provides lasting immunity
E   immunization is contraindicated in pregnancy

7   Pityriasis versicolor
A   is produced by the organism *Malassezia furfur*
B   is readily identified under ultraviolet light
C   is characteristically asymptomatic
D   typically produces lesions on the face and hands
E   responds to topical clotrimazole

8   An enterotoxin-mediated diarrhoea is produced by
A   *Staphylococcus aureus*
B   *Escherichia coli*
C   *Vibrio cholera*
D   *Shigella sonnei*
E   *Clostridium difficile*

9   The diagnosis of Weil's disease (leptospirosis) is confirmed by
A   liver biopsy
B   urine cultures
C   blood cultures
D   specific skin tests
E   serum antibody levels

10   Anthrax
A   is produced by a Gram-negative organism
B   has an incubation period of at least 2 weeks
C   produces a painful cutaneous abscess
D   is a common disease of animals in the UK
E   treatment is parenteral benzyl penicillin

11   In schistosomiasis
A   *Schistosoma haematobium* eggs inhabit the mesenteric veins of infected humans
B   the eggs of *Schistosoma japonicum* are passed in the faeces of infected individuals
C   the fresh water snail is the intermediate host of the *Schistosoma* species
D   bowel involvement can be diagnosed by rectal biopsy
E   oxamniquine is effective against all three species of worm

6	A	**False**	
	B	**True**	
	C	**True**	
	D	**True**	
	E	**True**	immunization is contraindicated during pregnancy; seronegative mothers should be immunized early in the post-partum period

7	A	**True**	the mycelial form of the commensal yeast *Pityrosporum orbiculare*
	B	**True**	it is more easily seen under Wood's light, giving a golden brown fluorescence
	C	**True**	
	D	**False**	skin lesions are usually on the trunk
	E	**True**	.

8	A	**True**	
	B	**True**	
	C	**True**	
	D	**False**	*Shigella sonnei* produces an enterotoxin that does not induce diarrhoea
	E	**True**	

9　A **False**　| the diagnosis can be established by blood
　　B **True**　| culture in the first week and urine culture
　　C **True**　⎬ in the second and third week. From the
　　D **False**　| second week onwards there is a rising titre
　　E **True**　| of specific leptospiral antibodies

10	A	**False**	anthrax is caused by a large aerobic Gram-positive bacillus
	B	**False**	the incubation period is 1–3 days
	C	**False**	the characteristic lesion is a necrotic or malignant pustule which is painless
	D	**False**	vaccination has virtually eliminated anthrax in animals in the UK
	E	**True**	treatment is with 1–2 megaunits of benzyl penicillin daily for 7 days

11	A	**False**	*Schistosoma haematobium* lives in the bladder, prostatic and uterine veins. *S. mansoni* and *S. japonicum* inhabit the mesenteric veins
	B	**True**	
	C	**True**	
	D	**True**	
	E	**False**	effective only against *S. mansoni*

12 In intestinal infections
A   *Campylobacter jejuni* is transmitted in infected milk and poultry
B   *Staphylococcus aureus* food poisoning usually produces vomiting within 6 hours of ingestion
C   *Vibrio parahaemolyticus* characteristically originates from seafood
D   salmonellosis usually produces diarrhoea within 12 hours
E   disseminated intravascular coagulation is a recognized complication of shigellosis

13 Human immunoglobulin is available for the passive immunization of
A   hepatitis B
B   measles
C   botulism
D   herpes zoster
E   diphtheria

14 Griseofulvin is
A   better absorbed after fatty meals
B   effective when used topically
C   most effective against the dermatophytes
D   ineffective in *Candida* infections
E   best given for many weeks in nail infections

15 *Mycobacterium leprae*
A   is best cultured on blood agar
B   is transmitted by the *Aedes* mosquito
C   is usually sensitive to rifampicin
D   bacteria are present in large numbers in tuberculoid leprosy
E   initial resistance to dapsone therapy is common

16 Recognized features of infection with *Salmonella typhi* include
A   maculopapular rash
B   splenomegaly
C   constipation
D   acute cholecystitis
E   neutropenia

12 A **True**
 B **True**
 C **True**
 D **False** salmonellosis usually produces diarrhoea in 12–24 hours
 E **True**

13 A **True** a specific hepatitis B immunoglobulin is available in association with vaccine
 B **True** human normal immunoglobulin is given
 C **True**
 D **True** specific varicella-zoster immunoglobulin is indicated in immunosuppressed patients at risk
 E **False** horse antitoxin is available

14 A **True**
 B **False**
 C **True**
 D **True**
 E **True** infections of nails require up to 12 months' treatment

15 A **False** cannot be grown on laboratory media
 B **False** there is no animal reservoir or proven insect vector
 C **True**
 D **False** the bacteria are present in low numbers in tuberculoid (paucibacillary) and large numbers in lepromatous (multibacillary) leprosy
 E **False** *M. leprae* is usually sensitive to dapsone

16 A **True** a 'rose-spot' maculopapular rash and splenomegaly are common during the second week of the illness
 B **True**
 C **True** constipation is frequent and more common than diarrhoea
 D **True** the gall bladder is frequently involved and may present as acute cholecystitis
 E **True** a common feature

17   Typical features of *Toxocara canis* infection include
A   unilateral visual impairment
B   eosinophilia
C   hepato-splenomegaly
D   subclinical infection
E   prompt response of ocular disease to diethylcarbamazine

18   Parasites which infect by direct cutaneous penetration include
A   *Necator americanus*
B   *Enterobius vermicularis*
C   *Ascaris lumbricoides*
D   *Ancylostoma duodenale*
E   *Strongyloides stercoralis*

19   A combination of at least two antibacterial agents are usually required to successfully treat
A   streptococcal pharyngitis
B   miliary tuberculosis
C   syphilis
D   enterococcal endocarditis
E   septicaemia in an immunosuppressed patient

20   Hepatitis B viral infection
A   has a carrier rate higher in females than in males
B   produces regular epidemics
C   is transmissible by sexual intercourse
D   is transmissible transplacentally to the fetus
E   human immunoglobulin gives up to 6 months' protection

21   Chickenpox
A   is caused by the same virus as herpes zoster
B   has an incubation period of 3–5 days
C   characteristically produces a centrifugal rash
D   rash exhibits cropping with lesions in various stages of maturation
E   pneumonia is commoner in adults than in children

22   In African trypanosomiasis
A   tsetse flies are the vectors of transmission
B   an inflamed bite site with regional lymphadenopathy is an early feature
C   the parasite can be readily seen in the peripheral blood film in the Gambian form of the disease
D   meningoencephalitis is typically late in rhodesiense infection
E   CNS changes indicate the need for suramin therapy

17 A **True**   the usual symptom of ocular toxocariasis
    B **True**
    C **True**   this is main physical sign in visceral larvae migrans
    D **True**   the majority of infections are subclinical
    E **False** the larvae are already dead

18 A **True**   ⎫ skin-penetrating parasites include the
                  hookworms *Necator americanus* and
    B **False** *Ancylostoma duodenale* and the intestinal
                  nematode, *Strongyloides stercoralis.*
    C **False** *Enterobius vermicularis* (threadworm) and
    D **True**   *Ascaris lumbricoides* (roundworm) are ingested
    E **True**   ⎭ by the victim

19 A **False** streptococcal pharyngitis and syphilis are best
                  treated with penicillin therapy alone
    B **True**   combined therapy is standard in tuberculosis
    C **False**
    D **True**
    E **True**

20 A **False** the carrier rate is 2–3 times higher in males than in
                  females
    B **False** hepatitis A occurs in epidemic form
    C **True**
    D **True**   chronic carriers commonly transmit the infection to
                  their babies, usually not transplacentally
    E **False** human immunoglobulin is relatively ineffective in
                  hepatitis B, unlike hepatitis A

21 A **True**
    B **False** the incubation period is 14–18 days
    C **False** the rash is characteristically centripetal and exhibits
                  cropping
    D **True**
    E **True**

22 A **True**
    B **True**   a trypanosomal chancre, the earliest sign, is present
                  in about 30%
    C **False** suggests Rhodesian form of the disease
    D **False** disease progresses rapidly in the Rhodesian form
                  and slowly in the Gambian form
    E **False** suramin does not pass the blood–brain barrier

23   Transmission by the faeco-oral route is usual in
   A   tularaemia
   B   ascariasis
   C   hepatitis A
   D   cysticercosis
   E   giardiasis

24   In tetanus infections
   A   clouding of consciousness is a typical feature
   B   a rigid abdomen is an early sign
   C   antitoxin neutralizes tetanus toxin within the central nervous system
   D   tetanic spasms indicate a poor prognosis
   E   survivors have life-long immunity

25   An incubation period of less than 7 days is a characteristic feature of
   A   mumps
   B   chickenpox
   C   diphtheria
   D   whooping cough
   E   anthrax

26   Characteristic features of the AIDS related complex (ARC) include
   A   a low CD4 lymphocyte count
   B   lymphadenopathy without other abnormality
   C   cerebral lymphoma
   D   diarrhoea
   E   weight loss

27   In food poisoning due to *Campylobacter jejuni*
   A   an enterotoxin is characteristically involved
   B   vomiting and abdominal pain occur within 6 hours of ingestion
   C   bloody diarrhoea is unusual
   D   clindamycin is the antibiotic of choice
   E   the organism is usually isolated from stools

28   Metronidazole is the treatment of choice in
   A   tularaemia
   B   South American trypanosomiasis (Chagas' disease)
   C   ancylostomiasis
   D   amoebiasis
   E   giardiasis

23 A **False**
B **True**
C **True**
D **False**
E **True**

tularaemia (*Francisella tularensis*) is usually spread by ticks or deerfly or ingestion of infected animal tissue. Cysticercosis is usually contracted from infected pork

---

24 A **False** the characteristic feature is mental alertness
B **True** common early signs include abdominal pain, dysphagia and stiffness in the jaw and back
C **False**
D **True** increases the risk of dying 25-fold
E **False** survivors require active immunization

---

25 A **False** 12–21 days, normally 18 days
B **False** 14–21 days
C **True**
D **False** 7–10 days, normally 7 days
E **True**

---

26 A **True**
B **False** weight loss, fever, diarrhoea and candidiasis are main features
C **False** this is full-blown AIDS
D **True**
E **True**

---

27 A **False** tissue-damaging bacteria rather than toxin producer
B **False** usually 12–48 hours after ingestion
C **False** a common feature
D **False** antibiotics required only for severe infection and choice would be ciprofloxacin or erythromycin
E **True**

---

28 A **False** streptomycin is most effective
B **False** nifurtimox and benzonidazole will clear blood of parasites in acute phase but do not offer radical cure
C **False** mebendazole is effective in hookworm infestation
D **True**
E **True**

29   Characteristic features of acute brucellosis include
  A   neutrophilic leucocytosis
  B   haemolytic anaemia
  C   backache
  D   profuse sweating
  E   prompt response to benzyl penicillin therapy

30   In diphtheria
  A   carriers should be treated with erythromycin
  B   primary infection can occur in the conjunctiva
  C   palatal palsy develops after laryngeal involvement
  D   antitoxin should be given after bacteriological confirmation
  E   cardiac conduction is impaired due to direct invasion of vagus nerve

31   In adult mumps infection
  A   unilateral orchitis is a recognized complication
  B   a macular rash is characteristic
  C   encephalitis is often fatal
  D   virus can be isolated from the cerebro-spinal fluid in lymphocytic meningitis
  E   abdominal pain usually indicates salpingo-oophoritis

32   Lyme disease
  A   is caused by tick-borne *Borrelia burgdorferi*
  B   is characterized by erythema chronicum migrans
  C   responds to treatment with intravenous penicillin
  D   results in septic arthritis
  E   is a recognized cause of cardiac conduction abnormalities

33   In *Plasmodium falciparum* malaria
  A   intermittent fever is characteristic
  B   ring forms of the parasite are seen on the blood film at an early stage
  C   hypoglycaemia is exacerbated by quinine treatment
  D   exchange transfusion is indicated if greater than 15% of erythrocytes are infected
  E   pregnancy enhances immunity to the disease

34   Useful drugs in the treatment of severe falciparum malaria include
  A   quinidine
  B   halofantrine
  C   chloroquine
  D   mefloquine
  E   proguanil

29 A **False** neutropenia with lymphocytosis
    B **False**
    C **True**
    D **True**
    E **False** doxycycline with rifampicin is optimal therapy

30 A **True**
    B **True**
    C **False** occurs about 10 days after <u>pharyngeal</u> or tonsillar diphtheria
    D **False** should be given immediately on clinical suspicion
    E **False** myocarditis causes conduction problems

31 A **True**
    B **False**
    C **False** the majority of patients recover completely
    D **True**
    E **False** pancreatitis is the more likely cause

32 A **True**
    B **True** this is a red macule or papule expanding to annular lesion—the 'bull's eye' lesion
    C **True**
    D **False** the recurrent asymmetrical arthritis is immunologically mediated
    E **True**

33 A **True**
    B **True** unlike other malarias when all stages of the life cycle are seen
    C **True** may give diagnostic difficulties in comatose patient
    D **True** can be life-saving
    E **False** immunity is impaired and parasitaemia frequently causes abortion

34 A **False** quinine not quinidine is used
    B **True** but contraindicated in pregnancy
    C **False** most strains chloroquine resistant
    D **True**
    E **False** used in chemoprophylaxis but not treatment

35   **In the UK compulsory notification of infectious diseases is required in cases of**
A   shigellosis
B   brucellosis
C   Legionnaire's disease
D   pertussis
E   AIDS

36   **Characteristic features of infection with *Pneumocystis carinii* in patients with AIDS include**
A   normal chest examination
B   weight loss
C   satisfactory response to nebulized pentamidine
D   interstitial shadowing on the chest X-ray
E   positive sputum cytology

37   **Respiratory symptoms are recognized clinical features in**
A   giardiasis
B   Rocky Mountain spotted fever
C   strongyloidiasis
D   onchocerciasis
E   ascariasis

38   **Recognized gastrointestinal manifestations of HIV infection include**
A   cytomegalovirus oesophagitis
B   *Helicobacter pylori* gastritis
C   cryptosporidial diarrhoea
D   microsporidiosis
E   small bowel lymphoma

39   **Recognized features of acquired toxoplasmosis include**
A   regional lymphadenopathy
B   sore throat
C   choroidoretinitis
D   necrotizing brain cyst
E   normal titres of IgG antibodies in adult uveitis

40   **Acyclovir is a useful agent in the treatment of**
A   respiratory syncitial virus infection
B   recurrent genital herpes simplex infection
C   sight-threatening cytomegalovirus infection
D   systemic varicella-zoster infection
E   herpes simplex encephalitis

35 A **True**   amoebic and bacillary dysentery are also notifiable
    B **False**
    C **False**
    D **True**
    E **False**   voluntary confidential reporting is encouraged

36 A **True**   must be suspected if weight loss, fever and
                   breathlessness occur
    B **True**
    C **True**   along with supportive therapy, including ventilation
    D **True**
    E **True**

37 A **False**   diarrhoea
    B **False**   rash, subcutaneous haemorrhages and
                   hepatosplenomegaly
    C **True**   wheezing and pneumonia
    D **False**   skin, lymph nodes and eyes (river blindness)
    E **True**   in migrating phase, pulmonary infiltrates can be
                   seen; symptoms are uncommon

38 A **True**   is a common cause of dysphagia
    B **False**   gastritis with hypochlorhydria is common but the
                   prevalence of infection with *H. pylori* is not increased
    C **True**
    D **True**   common cause of diarrhoea in the HIV-positive
                   patient
    E **True**

39 A **True**   seen in the asymptomatic adult
    B **False**
    C **True**   usually seen in congenital form, although rare in
                   acquired disease
    D **True**   especially in immunosuppressed patient
    E **True**   usually Sabin–Feldman dye test for IgG antibodies is
                   positive but can be negative in adult ocular disease

40 A **False**   tribavirin therapy
    B **True**
    C **False**   gancyclovir or foscarnet therapy
    D **True**
    E **True**

Endocrinology and metabolic disease

1 **Recognized complications of diabetes mellitus or its treatment include**
A pyoderma gangrenosum
B necrobiosis lipoidica diabeticorum
C lipohypertrophy
D moniliasis
E proximal myopathy

2 **Gynaecomastia occurs in association with**
A bronchogenic carcinoma
B spironolactone therapy
C XYY karyotype
D digoxin therapy
E Klinefelter's syndrome

3 **A man of 50 with weight loss and malaise of 6 months' duration has a serum sodium of 120 mmol/l. The following support a diagnosis of inappropriate ADH secretion**
A urinary osmolality persistently less than 300 mosmol/kg
B serum potassium 6 mmol/l
C nocturia and polyuria
D collapsed right upper lobe on chest X-ray
E blood urea 40 mmol/l

4 **A patient has a plasma potassium of 2.5 mmol/l and a plasma bicarbonate of 15 mmol/l. These findings are compatible with**
A renal tubular acidosis
B primary aldosteronism
C acute salicylate poisoning
D pyloric stenosis
E chronic respiratory failure

1 A **False**   a complication of ulcerative colitis
   B **True**   may predate diabetes
   C **True**   avoided by rotation of insulin injection sites
   D **True**
   E **False**   diabetics frequently develop a neuropathy

2 A **True**
   B **True**
   C **False**
   D **True**   especially in severe cardiac failure 'refeeding
                  gynaecomastia'
   E **True**   occurs in hypergonadotrophic hypogonadism

3 A **False**   urinary osmolality should be inappropriately high
                  given a low plasma osmolality
   B **False**   hyponatraemia stimulates aldosterone release;
                  serum potassium is usually normal or low
   C **False**   water is retained not excreted
   D **True**   small-cell lung carcinoma is the commonest cause
   E **False**   plasma osmolality and blood urea are low

4 A **True**
   B **False**   an alkalosis is associated with hypokalaemia
   C **True**
   D **False**   an alkalosis due to acid losses in urine and vomit
   E **False**   chronic respiratory acidosis results in compensated
                  metabolic alkalosis

5   **In thyrotoxicosis**
   A   carbimazole inhibits the uptake of plasma iodide into the thyroid gland
   B   a retrosternal goitre is a contraindication to radio-iodine therapy
   C   the diagnosis is confirmed by an elevated total T4
   D   the eye signs correlate poorly with the degree of thyrotoxicosis
   E   propranolol increases peripheral conversion of T4 to T3

6   **In normal growth**
   A   thyroxine is essential for cell maturation
   B   'bone age' correlates better with height than with weight
   C   enlargement of the testes is an early sign of puberty
   D   enlargement of the breasts is an early sign of puberty in girls
   E   gynaecomastia in a boy at puberty suggest the chromosomal composition is likely to be 47 XXY

7   **The following features help to distinguish chronic hypopituitarism from anorexia nervosa**
   A   decreased skin pigmentation
   B   amenorrhoea
   C   decreased body hair
   D   a lowered plasma cortisol level
   E   normal body fat

8   **Hypoglycaemia is a recognized feature in**
   A   Addison's disease
   B   acromegaly
   C   uraemia
   D   hepatocellular failure
   E   chronic pancreatitis

9   **Recognized findings in primary hypothyroidism include**
   A   coma
   B   cerebellar ataxia
   C   intestinal obstruction
   D   pericardial effusion
   E   increased cholesterol synthesis

5 A **False** carbimazole blocks iodination of tyrosine
   B **False** not a contraindication; surgery may be more appropriate
   C **False** elevated free T4 and low TSH
   D **True**   exophthalmos may predate thyrotoxicosis; in the elderly, eye signs are often absent
   E **False** propranolol reduces peripheral T4 conversion to T3

6 A **True**   thyroxine is necessary for normal growth
   B **True**   there is more variation in weight than height in any group of individuals
   C **True**   the earliest sign in most boys
   D **True**   the earliest sign in most girls
   E **False** gynaecomastia is normal in boys at puberty

7 A **True**   pallor is a striking feature of hypopituitarism
   B **False** amenorrhoea is a diagnostic feature of both conditions
   C **True**   patients with anorexia nervosa have increased body hair (lanugo)
   D **True**   adrenal function is normal in anorexia nervosa
   E **True**   loss of body fat occurs in anorexia nervosa

8 A **True**   cortisol is an insulin antagonist
   B **False** growth hormone is an insulin antagonist
   C **True**   especially in patients treated with beta-blockers on haemodialysis
   D **True**   absence of liver glycogen
   E **True**   usually hyperglycaemia, though hypoglycaemia can occur on rare occasions

9 A **True**   especially if hypothermic
   B **True**
   C **True**   a visceral myopathy
   D **True**
   E **False** the elevated plasma cholesterol is probably due to decreased utilization

10 Features of primary hypoparathyroidism include
A paraesthesia
B abnormal calcification on skull X-ray
C associated peptic ulceration
D cataracts
E metacarpal abnormalities

11 In Klinefelter's syndrome
A the testes are small
B mental retardation is usual
C plasma FSH is normal
D sperm production is normal
E the sex chromosomes show 47 XYY

12 In a 21-year-old young woman complaining of 18 months' weakness, constipation, polyuria and polydipsia not associated with weight loss
A polyuria due to diabetes mellitus cannot be excluded by urinalysis alone
B serum calcium should be measured
C analgesic intake should be assessed
D a previous history of erythema nodosum is relevant
E the most likely diagnosis is compulsive water drinking

13 In primary hyperparathyroidism
A serum phosphate is characteristically elevated
B urinary phosphate excretion is reduced
C serum calcium rises in response to treatment with thiazide diuretics
D the prevalence in the community is about 1:1000
E in the young patient, surgery is indicated only if symptoms persist

14 In Cushing's disease
A urinary free cortisol excretion is invariably elevated
B X-rays of the pituitary fossa are usually abnormal
C hypertension is a characteristic feature
D negative nitrogen balance is characteristic
E treatment with trilostane is effective

10	A	**True**	due to tetany
	B	**True**	basal ganglia calcification
	C	**False**	
	D	**True**	occurs in 50% of cases
	E	**False**	the pseudohypoparathyroid syndromes

11	A	**True**	classical feature
	B	**False**	intelligence usually preserved although retardation is a rare finding
	C	**False**	hypergonadotrophic hypogonadism
	D	**False**	no spermatozoa are produced
	E	**False**	47 XXY

12	A	**False**	polyuria in diabetes is due to the osmotic diuresis and glycosuria will be detected
	B	**True**	hypercalcaemia causes a picture identical to nephrogenic diabetes insipidus
	C	**True**	this may be renal failure due to analgesic nephropathy
	D	**True**	renal sarcoidosis or diabetes insipidus from cerebral sarcoid should be considered
	E	**True**	

13	A	**False**	the serum phosphate is low
	B	**False**	urinary phosphate excretion enhanced
	C	**True**	thiazide diuretics may precipitate hypercalcaemia
	D	**True**	
	E	**False**	asymptomatic individuals under 50 should have neck exploration

14	A	**True**	on rare occasions, disease activity is episodic
	B	**False**	the X-rays of the pituitary fossa are usually normal (65% cases)
	C	**True**	
	D	**True**	corticosteroids are catabolic hormones
	E	**True**	3β-hydroxyenzyme inhibitor that blocks cortisol synthesis

15   Amenorrhoea is a typical finding in
   A   the Stein–Leventhal syndrome
   B   profound weight loss
   C   Sheehan's syndrome
   D   acute stress reactions
   E   Turner's syndrome

16   Oral hypoglycaemic drugs
   A   should be avoided in diabetics with a history of ketoacidosis
   B   sulphonylurea drugs have a more potent hypoglycaemic action than metformin
   C   should be withdrawn during pregnancy
   D   metformin causes lactic acidosis
   E   are indicated after total pancreatectomy

17   In acromegaly
   A   visual field defects are an indication for external irradiation
   B   excessive sweating is a typical symptom
   C   hypocalciuria is an expected finding
   D   hypopituitarism requires exclusion during follow-up
   E   the underlying tumour is usually a chromophobe adenoma

18   Hyperthyroidism is a recognized association in
   A   pituitary tumours
   B   choriocarcinoma
   C   testicular terato-carcinoma
   D   iodide therapy
   E   differentiated thyroid carcinoma

19   Normal puberty is characterised
   A   by scrotal rugosity as a first feature in boys
   B   by growth of pubic hair as a first feature in girls
   C   by an average age of menarche of 15 years in the UK
   D   by pubic hair appearing before enlargement of the testes
   E   by menstruation usually occurring after breast development is completed

15 A **False** oligomenorrhoea usually
    B **True**
    C **True**   hypopituitarism
    D **True**
    E **True**   karyotype 45, XO gonadal dysgenesis

16 A **True**   DKA usually indicates insulin dependency
    B **True**   hypoglycaemia never occurs with metformin alone
    C **True**   all diabetics who are pregnant should have insulin
    D **True**   especially if renal or hepatic impairment is present
    E **False** exogenous insulin is required

17 A **False** surgery is indicated if visual field defects are found
    B **True**
    C **False** hypercalciuria in 50%
    D **True**   especially in large tumours
    E **False** usually eosinophil adenoma

18 A **True** ⎫
    B **True** ⎬ rare
    C **True** ⎭
    D **True**   Jod–Basedow phenomenon
    E **True**   only if metastases are extensive

19 A **True**
    B **False** breast development occurs first
    C **False** the average age is 13
    D **False** testicular enlargement occurs first
    E **False** menstruation is invariably established before breast
                  development is complete

20   Recognized causes of hyperprolactinaemia include
A   hypothyroidism
B   craniopharyngioma
C   cimetidine therapy
D   metoclopramide therapy
E   oral contraceptive therapy

21   Characteristic features of chronic adrenocortical insufficiency include
A   weight loss
B   nocturia
C   diarrhoea
D   glycosuria
E   depression

22   Weight loss is a characteristic feature of
A   diabetes insipidus
B   hyperparathyroidism
C   Addison's disease
D   acromegaly
E   phaeochromocytoma

23   Non-metastatic complications of malignant disease include
A   parathyroid hormone-like activity in squamous bronchial carcinomas
B   calcitonin secretion by bronchial carcinomas
C   chorionic gonadotrophin secretion by hepatoblastomas
D   adrenocorticotrophic hormone secretion by gastric carcinomas
E   antidiuretic hormone secretion by pancreatic carcinoma

24   In congenital adrenal hyperplasia of the 21-hydroxylase type
A   inheritance is autosomal recessive
B   the diagnosis is confirmed by elevated plasma levels of 17 hydroxyprogesterone
C   on presentation there is usually evidence of adrenal insufficiency
D   the condition presents as testicular hypertrophy in males
E   ambiguous genitalia is a characteristic feature in neonates

20 A **True** ⎫
    B **True** ⎪
    C **True** ⎬ and galactorrhoea may also occur
    D **True** ⎪
    E **True** ⎭

21 A **True**   usually 5–15 kg
    B **True**   renal tubular dysfunction
    C **True**   GI disturbance is one of the main symptoms
    D **False**
    E **True**   psychiatric disturbance is often seen

22 A **False** patients drink to make up water loss
    B **False**
    C **True**   characteristically due to anorexia
    D **False**
    E **True**   anorexia, sympathetic overdrive and impaired
                   glucose tolerance all contribute

23 A **True**   the only hormone not commonly produced by small-
                   cell carcinomas
    B **True**   but no actual clinical syndrome
    C **True**   in children
    D **True**   rare
    E **True**

24 A **True**   most enzyme defects are autosomal recessive
    B **True**   17 hydroxyprogesterone is formed before enzyme
                   block
    C **True**   characteristic
    D **True**   macrogenitosomia in the male infant is characteristic
    E **True**   if female with an XX karyotype

25 **Urinary delta aminolaevulinic acid and porphobilinogen are characteristically elevated in**
    A   acute intermittent porphyria
    B   porphyria cutanea tarda
    C   porphyria variegata
    D   erythropoietic uroporphyria
    E   erythropoietic protoporphyria

26 **In toxic multinodular goitre**
    A   free T4 is elevated and the TSH is normal
    B   carbimazole therapy is ineffective
    C   exophthalmos is more common than in Graves' disease
    D   thyroid microsomal antibodies are present in high titres
    E   thyroid calcification on neck X-rays is common

27 **In anorexia nervosa**
    A   plasma cortisol levels are decreased
    B   plasma growth hormone levels are increased
    C   the male/female ratio affected is 1:3
    D   plasma gonadotrophins are normal
    E   plasma TSH levels are normal

28 **In diabetic retinopathy**
    A   microaneurysms are pathognomonic of the condition
    B   visual acuity is usually preserved in exudative maculopathy
    C   neovascularization around the optic disc is a pre-proliferative feature
    D   colour blindness is a characteristic development
    E   argon laser photocoagulation is difficult in the presence of cataract

29 **Phaeochromocytomas**
    A   are found in 5% of hypertensive patients
    B   are multiple in 50% of patients
    C   are locally malignant in 10% of cases
    D   produce noradrenaline particularly in adrenal tumours
    E   are best diagnosed by the phentolamine test

25 A **True**   in both acute and latent phase
    B **False**   but are elevated in congenital hepatic porphyria
    C **True**
    D **False** ⎫
    E **False** ⎭ both are normal

26 A **False**   TSH is suppressed and free T4 elevated
    B **False**   medical and surgical therapy are equally effective
    C **False**   exophthalmos is more common in Graves' disease
    D **False**   Graves' disease
    E **True**

27 A **False**   usually normal
    B **True**
    C **False**   10- to 20-fold increase in females
    D **False**   usually suppressed
    E **True**

28 A **False**   can be seen in haematological conditions
    B **False**   this is a symptomatic diabetic retinopathy
    C **False**   this is proliferative feature
    D **False**
    E **True**   cataracts sometimes require removal first

29 A **False**   less than 0.1% of hypertensives
    B **False**   about 10% are multiple
    C **True**
    D **True**   more so than adrenaline
    E **False**   plasma noradrenaline estimation and CT scanning

30   Radiological changes in osteomalacia include
   A   stress fractures of metatarsals
   B   multilocular bone cysts
   C   decreased bone density in the lateral scapular margins
   D   subperiosteal bone resorption
   E   biconcave vertebrae

31   The following disorders are associated with impaired carbohydrate tolerance
   A   Friedreich's ataxia
   B   Down's syndrome
   C   Klinefelter's syndrome
   D   Sippel's syndrome (MEN type II)
   E   Huntington's chorea

32   Antidiuretic hormone secretion is stimulated by
   A   ethyl alcohol
   B   reduction in plasma volume
   C   increased plasma osmolality
   D   acute stress
   E   morphine administration

33   Recognized features of haemochromatosis include
   A   melanin deposits in the skin
   B   hypoglycaemia
   C   testicular atrophy
   D   equal incidence of homozygotes for the haemochromatosis gene in men and women
   E   HLA A_3 positive in 70% of patients

34   Complications of fulminant diabetic ketoacidosis or its treatment include
   A   pneumomediastinum
   B   permanent cataracts
   C   myocarditis
   D   cerebral oedema
   E   acquired respiratory distress syndrome (ARDS)

30	A	**True**	
	B	**False**	a feature of hyperparathyroidism
	C	**True**	Looser's zones
	D	**False**	osteoporosis and hyperparathyroidism
	E	**True**	'codfish' vertebrae

31	A	**True**	10% have diabetes
	B	**True**	
	C	**False**	
	D	**True**	this is phaeochromocytoma, medullary carcinoma of thyroid and parathyroid hyperplasia
	E	**True**	

32	A	**False**	ADH secretion is inhibited by a rising blood alcohol level
	B	**True**	
	C	**True**	
	D	**True**	
	E	**True**	central effect. Also stimulated by nausea

33	A	**True**	associated with increased iron deposits
	B	**False**	diabetes occurs in 80% of cases
	C	**True**	a combination of testicular and pituitary impairment
	D	**True**	more severe disease in males
	E	**True**	

34	A	**True**	pneumomediastinum may result from severe vomiting and retching
	B	**False**	long-term complication of diabetes
	C	**False**	
	D	**True**	induced by inappropriate hypotonic fluid therapy
	E	**True**	

35 In medullary carcinoma of the thyroid gland
 A secretory products include prostaglandins, ACTH, serotonin and calcitonin
 B there is an equal incidence in males and females
 C a 'hot' spot area is seen on the thyroid scan
 D the treatment of choice is high-dose radio-iodine
 E distal metastases are usual at presentation

36 Elevation of the plasma alkaline phosphatase is a typical finding in
 A homocystinuria
 B Paget's disease
 C hypophosphatasia
 D osteomalacia
 E osteogenesis imperfecta

37 Diabetes mellitus is associated with
 A primary hyperaldosteronism (Conn's syndrome)
 B acromegaly
 C glucagonoma
 D cystic fibrosis
 E acanthosis nigricans

38 In an attack of acute intermittent porphyria
 A photosensitivity is a characteristic feature
 B plasma porphobilinogen (PBG) is characteristically elevated
 C pregnancy is a recognized precipitating factor
 D urinary levels of delta-aminolaevulinate (ALA) are elevated
 E seizures should be treated with carbamazepine therapy

35 A **True**
    B **True**   unlike other thyroid cancer with a female
                   preponderance
    C **False**   a cold area
    D **False**   iodine is not taken up by parafollicular C cells—total
                   thyroidectomy is indicated
    E **True**

36 A **False**   alkaline phosphatase is normal
    B **True**
    C **False**   alkaline phosphatase is low
    D **True**   usually but not always elevated
    E **False**   alkaline phosphatase is normal

37 A **False**
    B **True**   glucagon and growth hormone are insulin
                   antagonists
    C **True**
    D **True**   diabetes may be a presenting feature in older
                   children
    E **True**   rare abnormality of insulin receptors

38 A **False**   but seen in most other porphyrias
    B **True**   contributing to acute neurological, psychiatric and GI
                   disturbance
    C **True**
    D **True**   increased delta ALA synthetase activity
    E **False**   diazepam or valproate is safer

39 In type 1 diabetes mellitus
    A there is an association with HLA DR3 and DR4
    B glucagon and somatostatin secretion is normal
    C complement fixing islet cell antibodies are typically present
    D concordance in monozygotic twins is about 90%
    E insulin receptor antibodies enhance insulin sensitivity

40 Recognized features of diabetic neuropathy include
    A foot ulcers that are typically painless
    B unilateral upper abdominal pain
    C amyotrophy resolving with improved glycaemic control
    D impotence that responds to intracavernosal papaveretum
    E preservation of temperature sensation

39 A **True**
    B **True**   at diagnosis only beta cells are affected, with alpha
                   and delta cell function preserved
    C **True**
    D **False**   around 50%
    E **False**   cause insulin resistance

40 A **True**
    B **True**   diabetic radiculopathy
    C **True**
    D **False**   intracavernosal papaverine
    E **False**   pain and temperature sensation soon become
                   abnormal

Nephrology

1 **In adult polycystic disease of the kidney**
   A renal dialysis is usually necessary by the age of 20 years
   B cysts involve all parts of the nephron
   C proteinuria of 4 g per day is an expected finding
   D intracerebral aneurysms are a recognized association
   E the abnormal gene is detected on chromosome 16

2 **A urine osmolality of 360 mosmol/kg with a urine sodium of 50 mmol/l is an expected finding in**
   A pre-renal uraemia due to dehydration
   B acute oliguric renal failure
   C acute non-oliguric renal failure
   D acute obstructive uropathy
   E acute post-streptococcal glomerulonephritis

3 **Early findings in post-streptococcal glomerulonephritis include**
   A dyspnoea
   B convulsions
   C oliguria with a urine sodium concentration of less than
      12 mmol/l
   D glomerular epithelial crescents
   E red cell casts in the urine

4 **Under normal conditions, glomerular filtration rate is primarily regulated by**
   A glomerular capillary pressure
   B intracapsular hydrostatic pressure
   C renal prostaglandin synthesis
   D plasma colloid oncotic pressure
   E juxtaglomerular apparatus aldosterone production

5 **Hypocomplementaemia and glomerulonephritis are recognized features of**
   A bacterial endocarditis
   B systemic lupus erythematosus
   C polyarteritis nodosa
   D Goodpasture's syndrome
   E membranous glomerulonephritis

1 A **False** renal failure may be delayed past the age of 45 years
   B **True**
   C **False**
   D **True**   occur in 20% of patients
   E **True**   genetic counselling is advisable

2 A **False** urine sodium is classically below 10 mmol/l and
                 urine osmolality is elevated
   B **True** ⎱ tubular dysfunction prevents sodium re-absorption
   C **True** ⎰ and leads to an inappropriately high urine sodium
   D **True**
   E **False**

3 A **True**   convulsions and dyspnoea are manifestations of
                 severe hypertension which develops rapidly when
                 associated with glomerular crescent formation
   B **True**
   C **True**   if there is no tubular dysfunction, sodium re-
                 absorption is normal
   D **True** ⎱ characteristic
   E **True** ⎰

4 A **True**
   B **False**
   C **False** only influences GFR under stressed conditions
   D **False**
   E **False** JGA produces renin

5 A **True**   complement levels are often, but not invariably,
                 depressed in subacute bacterial endocarditis and
                 systemic lupus erythematosus
   B **True**
   C **False** ⎤
   D **False** ⎬ normal serum complement
   E **False** ⎦

6   Goodpasture's syndrome
   A   is associated with highly-selective proteinuria
   B   should be treated with plasmapheresis and/or cytotoxic
        therapy
   C   typically presents with severe dyspnoea
   D   is a soluble-complex type of nephritis
   E   is often associated with neurological features at presentation

7   Acute nephritic presentation is a characteristic feature of
   A   mesangiocapillary glomerulonephritis
   B   end-stage renal failure
   C   minimal change glomerulonephritis
   D   systemic lupus erythematosus
   E   Behçet's disease

8   Renal calcification is a recognized feature of
   A   analgesic nephropathy
   B   medullary sponge kidney
   C   renal cortical necrosis
   D   sarcoidosis
   E   Fanconi's syndrome in adults

**9   In a woman with polyuria and polydipsia, compulsive water
     drinking is the likely diagnosis if**
   A   there is a previous history of psychiatric disorder
   B   symptoms are worse after intramuscular desmopressin
   C   the plasma osmolality is elevated
   D   water deprivation produces increased urine concentration
   E   there is a visual field defect

10   Proteinuria of more than 10 g/day is a recognized finding in
   A   diabetic nephropathy
   B   renal tubular necrosis
   C   chronic mercury poisoning
   D   adult Fanconi syndrome
   E   chronic pyelonephritis

11   Renal failure due to sarcoidosis occurs as a result of
   A   nephrolithiasis
   B   granulomatous nephropathy
   C   chronic glomerulonephritis
   D   obstructive uropathy
   E   minimal change glomerulonephritis

6 A **False** unselective proteinuria
     B **True**
     C **True** anaemia, dyspnoea, pulmonary haemorrhage and severe glomerulonephritis
     D **False** circulating antibody to renal and pulmonary basement membranes
     E **False**

---

7 A **True** acute nephritis presents with oliguria, haematuria, fluid retention and hypertension
     B **False**
     C **False** nephrotic syndrome
     D **True**
     E **False** only on rare occasions associated with a glomerulonephritis

---

8 A **True** papillary calcification
     B **True** in the pyramidal cysts
     C **True** develops many weeks after onset
     D **True** hypercalcaemia and hypercalciuria are typical
     E **False** proximal tubular defect with acidosis and osteomalacia

---

9 A **True** most frequently seen in psychoneurotic females
     B **True** water-intoxication develops if the patient continues to drink
     C **False** plasma osmolality is reduced
     D **True** reduction in urine volume and increase in urine concentration
     E **False** diabetes insipidus due to pituitary tumour

---

10 A **True**
      B **False**
      C **True** causes nephrotic syndrome
      D **False** uncommon in interstitial nephropathy
      E **False**

---

11 A **True** hypercalcaemia, hypercalciuria, nephrolithiasis and obstructive uropathy are the commonest renal manifestations of sarcoidosis but renal failure due to granulomatous infiltration and proliferative glomerulonephritis have been described
      B **True**
      C **True**
      D **True** ·
      E **False**

12 **The following adverse drug effects are associated with**
   A   amphotericin—glomerulonephritis
   B   penicillamine—Goodpasture's syndrome
   C   isoniazid—acute tubular necrosis
   D   demeclocycline—nephrogenic diabetes insipidus
   E   gold—membranous nephropathy

13 **Renal impairment in polyarteritis nodosa is caused by**
   A   ureteric strictures
   B   hypertension
   C   rapidly progressive proliferative glomerulonephritis
   D   interstitial nephritis
   E   minimal change glomerulonephritis

14 **Relative contraindications to ultrasound guided percutaneous renal biopsy include**
   A   platelet count of less than 50×10^9/l
   B   creatinine clearance 50 ml/minute
   C   absence of one kidney
   D   polyarteritis nodosa
   E   blood pressure 180/120

15 **Recognized findings in hereditary nephritis (Alport's syndrome) include**
   A   nerve deafness
   B   optic atrophy
   C   haematuria
   D   autosomal dominance
   E   prognosis worse in males

16 **Common causes of death among chronic haemodialysis patients, include**
   A   exsanguination
   B   cerebrovascular accident
   C   myocardial infarction
   D   systemic infection
   E   air embolism

12 A **False** amphotericin causes proximal and distal tubular damage
    B **True**   also renal vasculitis and membranous nephropathy
    C **False** drug-induced lupus syndrome
    D **True**   reversibly inhibits adenylate cyclase in collecting tubules
    E **True**   occurs in 1% of patients

13 A **True**   macroscopic PAN affects renal arcuate vessels and may cause severe hypertension and ureteric vasculitic lesions. Microscopic PAN causes rapidly progressive glomerulonephritis
    B **True**
    C **True**
    D **False**
    E **False**

14 A **True**   uncontrolled hypertension, thrombocytopenia, clotting disorders or the presence of only one kidney are absolute contraindications to percutaneous renal biopsy
    B **False**
    C **True**
    D **True**   arteriography may reveal the presence of micro-aneurysms in polyarteritis nodosa and the risk of haemorrhage is increased
    E **True**

15 A **True**   sensorineural deafness is characteristic
    B **False** lens abnormalities
    C **True**   platelet and renal glomerular basement membrane abnormalities
    D **True**   some families X-linked
    E **True**

16 A **False** deaths due to technical faults, e.g. exsanguination, air embolism, are rare
    B **True** ⎫ the death rate is approximately 10% per year,
    C **True** ⎬ due largely to the effects of atherosclerosis
    D **True** ⎭ and infection
    E **False**

17   In human renal transplantation
  A   a graft from an identical twin rarely produces rejection
  B   autografts should be used in preference to homografts
  C   homografts from close relatives are more successful than homografts from unrelated individuals
  D   cyclosporin is only required in the early post-operative phase
  E   anaemia is the commonest cause of death

18   Symptoms of an acute rejection episode following renal transplantation include
  A   peripheral oedema
  B   fever
  C   polyarthritis
  D   pain in the graft
  E   polyuria

19   In renal failure, peritoneal dialysis
  A   aids correction of acidosis and hyperkalaemia
  B   produces hyperglycaemia if hypertonic solutions are used
  C   should be used only in chronic renal failure
  D   aggravates hypoproteinaemia
  E   is useful in controlling hypertension

20   Recognized complications of renal transplantation include
  A   gallstones
  B   lymphoma
  C   avascular necrosis of bone
  D   widespread warts
  E   polycythaemia

21   In health, the kidney regulates the blood pH by the excretion of
  A   ammonia
  B   free hydrogen ions
  C   free organic acid
  D   sodium monohydrogen phosphate
  E   glutamine

17   A   **True**   almost 100% successful
     B   **False**   both kidneys are diseased for renal failure to occur
     C   **True**   homografts from relatives have the next best survival rates
     D   **False**   even with living related donor transplants, life-long immunosuppression is required to prevent rejection
     E   **False**   deaths are usually from infection and/or uncontrolled rejection; erythropoietin is useful in controlling anaemia

18   A   **True**   acute rejection decreases sodium excretion
     B   **True**
     C   **False**   manifestations may include hypertension and 'flu-like' symptoms
     D   **True**
     E   **False**   acute tubular necrosis is not uncommon but is not related to rejection

19   A   **True**
     B   **True**   dialysis solutions use glucose as an osmotic agent and hypertonic solutions may result in hyperglycaemia
     C   **False**
     D   **True**   dialysate protein losses can exceed 30 g/day
     E   **True**

20   A   **False**
     B   **True**   the incidence of non-Hodgkin's lymphomas is increased almost 60-fold by cytotoxic therapy
     C   **True**   particularly of the femoral heads due to cumulative steroid dosage
     D   **True**   in up to 40% of transplant patients due to immunosuppression
     E   **True**   in chronically rejecting transplants

21   A   **True**   excretion of ammonia, H^+ ions, organic acids and sodium monohydrogen phosphate are all involved in pH regulation by the kidney
     B   **True**
     C   **True**
     D   **True**
     E   **False**   glutamine is synthesized by the renal tubular cells and broken down to release ammonia for excretion

22 **A patient has a blood urea of 40 mmol/l, a normal blood pressure and kidneys of normal size and shape on renal ultrasound. These findings would be expected in**
A   congenital polycystic kidneys
B   myelomatosis
C   urinary tract infection
D   acute glomerulonephritis
E   analgesic nephropathy

23 **Haemodialysis is better than peritoneal dialysis in**
A   controlling hypercatabolic states
B   removing dialysable drugs
C   being tolerated by both young and old patients
D   avoiding respiratory failure
E   removing excess fluid efficiently

24 **A man of 30 was rejected for life insurance because of a blood pressure of 220/130. On examination, fundoscopy revealed narrowing of the retinal arteries, small soft retinal exudates and early papilloedema. The heart was not clinically enlarged, a systolic murmur was audible in the epigastrium and there was a large amount of urinary albumin on urine testing**
A   the evidence is insufficient to justify the diagnosis of accelerated hypertension
B   if excretion urography after 20 minutes shows a less dense shadow in the left renal pelvis, the presence of a left renal artery stenosis is likely
C   the *best* way of confirming renal artery stenosis is selective arteriography
D   if a patient with renal artery stenosis is treated surgically, a normal blood pressure immediately after the operation indicates permanent success in removing the cause of hypertension
E   hypokalaemia indicates an aldosterone-secreting tumour

25 **Recognized causes of the nephrotic syndrome include**
A   amyloidosis
B   Henoch–Schönlein purpura
C   renal vein thrombosis
D   gold therapy
E   minimal-change glomerulonephritis·

22 A **False** renal enlargement with asymmetrical outlines
    B **True**   renal amyloidosis
    C **False** UTI does not usually cause renal failure
    D **False** normal blood pressure would be unusual with acute
                  glomerulonephritis and renal impairment
    E **False** small, shrunken kidneys

23 A **True**   haemodialysis is more efficient than peritoneal
                  dialysis
    B **True**   with present techniques of ultrafiltration, the
                  removal of dialysable drugs and fluid is very efficient
    C **False** peritoneal dialysis is often better tolerated
    D **True**   respiratory problems are caused by limitation of
                  diaphragmatic movement
    E **True**

24 A **False** severe hypertension with evidence of end organ
                  damage (retinopathy and proteinuria)
    B **False** <u>dense</u> persistent nephrogram on the affected side
    C **True**
    D **False** the result of surgical treatment should be assessed 6
                  months post-operatively as recurrence is not
                  uncommon
    E **False** seen in accelerated hypertension due to secondary
                  hyperaldosteronism

25 A **True**   amyloid, Henoch–Schönlein purpura, gold therapy
                  and minimal change glomerulonephritis are all
                  recognized causes
    B **True**
    C **False** this is a result not cause and is a manifestation of the
                  increased thrombotic tendency seen in the nephrotic
                  syndrome
    D **True**
    E **True**

26   **In membranous glomerulonephritis**
    A the onset is typically acute
    B spontaneous remissions are common
    C macroscopic haematuria is characteristic
    D steroid therapy is contraindicated
    E a familial tendency is characteristic

27   **Typical features of acute tubular necrosis include**
    A red cell casts in the urine
    B granular casts in the urine
    C daily urine output 400 ml, osmolality 700 mosmol/kg
    D daily urine output 1200 ml, osmolality 310 mosmol/kg
    E absent renal perfusion on a technetium scan

28   **Findings of clinical significance in a urinary deposit include**
    A granular casts
    B red cell casts
    C magnesium ammonium phosphate crystals
    D visible bacilli on microscopy of uncentrifuged urine
    E mononuclear cells in centrifuged urine

29   **The plasma creatinine is**
    A lower in females than in males
    B elevated in the early stages of renal failure
    C lower in the elderly than in the young
    D accurately reflects the glomerular filtration rate in advanced renal failure
    E elevated in hypercatabolic states

30   **In acute renal failure, hyperkalaemia is**
    A usually symptomatic
    B aggravated by hypercatabolic states
    C characteristically associated with flat T waves on ECG
    D a medical emergency if levels rise above 6.5 mmol/l
    E usefully treated by oral cation-exchange resins

31   **A 50-year-old male presents with acute renal failure and jaundice. The following features are likely to be of clinical relevance**
    A keen inland-water sportsman
    B pre-existing alcoholism
    C tricyclic antidepressant therapy
    D paracetamol overdosage
    E lead exposure

26 A **False**   usually insidious onset
    B **False**   usually progresses to chronic renal failure
    C **False**
    D **False**   may benefit from steroids and chlorambucil therapy
    E **False**   although a few familial cases have been reported

27 A **False**   red cell casts indicate a proliferative
                   glomerulonephritis
    B **True**
    C **False**   ⎫ urine volume may be low or high and the urine and
                   ⎬ plasma iso-osmolar
    D **True**   ⎭
    E **False**   renal perfusion is normal or reduced

28 A **True**   granular and red cell casts are seen in
                   glomerulonephritis
    B **True**
    C **False**   normal finding
    D **True**   visible bacilli usually signify infection
    E **True**   important in detecting transplant rejection

29 A **True**   plasma creatinine is proportional to muscle mass
                   (lower in females and the elderly)
    B **False**   plasma creatinine may still be normal, despite
                   decreased creatinine clearance
    C **True**
    D **False**   tubular secretion of creatinine rises, leading to an
                   overestimate of renal function
    E **True**   increased muscle breakdown

30 A **False**
    B **True**   hyperkalaemia develops more rapidly in
                   hypercatabolic states
    C **False**   peaked T waves are indicative of hyperkalaemia
    D **True**   danger of cardiac standstill
    E **True**   causes increased potassium loss

31 A **True**   leptospirosis or Weil's disease
    B **True**   hepatorenal syndrome in advanced cirrhosis
    C **False**
    D **True**   characteristic in severe untreated overdoses
    E **True**   rare but hepatitis can occur

32   **A mentally retarded young woman with cataracts is found to have hypocalcaemia. Findings supporting a diagnosis of pseudohypoparathyroidism include**
   A   undetectable plasma PTH
   B   hyperphosphataemia
   C   no increase in urinary AMP excretion during vitamin D therapy
   D   impaired renal function
   E   skeletal and dental abnormalities

33   **In the anaemia of chronic renal failure**
   A   a normochromic normocytic blood film is characteristic
   B   folic acid supplementation is usually effective
   C   due to polycystic disease, anaemia is characteristically mild
   D   a rapid response to erythropoietin therapy is typical
   E   renal transplantation rarely improves anaemia

34   **Indications for the introduction of renal dialysis in chronic renal failure include**
   A   plasma creatinine greater than 500 μmol/l
   B   uraemic pericarditis
   C   persistent anaemia
   D   intractable acidosis
   E   proteinuria greater than 10 g/day

35   **Effective treatments in prostatic malignancy include**
   A   finasteride
   B   leuprorelin
   C   formestane
   D   spironolactone
   E   flutamide

36   **In diabetic nephropathy**
   A   an increased blood pressure is an early feature
   B   a high-protein diet is advised if proteinuria is severe
   C   insulin requirements fall in end-stage disease
   D   angiotensin-converting enzyme inhibitors reduce microalbuminuria
   E   renal transplantation is contraindicated if retinopathy is severe

37   **A low level of plasma magnesium is seen**
   A   in adrenocortical insufficiency
   B   with osteolytic bone metastases
   C   after surgical correction of hyperparathyroidism
   D   during cisplatin therapy
   E   in chronic alcoholism

32 A **False** high circulating PTH levels
    B **True**
    C **True** renal tubular insensitivity to PTH
    D **False** renal function is otherwise normal
    E **True**

33 A **True**
    B **False** haematinic therapy is ineffective
    C **True** erythropoietin is usually still made in polycystic disease
    D **True**
    E **False**

34 A **False** often ≥ 1000 μmol/l if clinically stable
    B **True**
    C **False** treatable with erythropoietin
    D **True**
    E **False** unusual in chronic renal failure

35 A **False** 5-alpha-reductase inhibitor useful in benign prostatic hypertrophy
    B **True** inhibitor of gonadotrophin-releasing hormone
    C **False** aromatase inhibitor which blocks conversion of androgens to oestrogens; used in advanced breast cancer
    D **False**
    E **True** an anti-androgen useful if GnRH inhibitors fail to control disease

36 A **False** occurs late in the disease
    B **False** lowering dietary protein intake decelerates progression
    C **True** increased insulin sensitivity
    D **True**
    E **False**

37 A **False** magnesium levels are usually normal
    B **True**
    C **True** 'hungry bones' syndrome; also magnesium and calcium compete for renal tubular excretion
    D **True** renal losses
    E **True** often parallels plasma potassium levels

38   Painless microscopic haematuria is a typical presenting feature of
A   IgA nephropathy
B   renal infarction
C   renal tuberculosis
D   multiple myeloma
E   mesangiocapillary glomerulonephritis

39   Hormones synthesized by the normal kidney include
A   parathormone
B   atrial natriuretic peptide
C   1,25-dihydroxy vitamin D
D   prostaglandin E_2
E   kallikrein

40   Radio-opaque renal stones include
A   calcium phosphate
B   cystine
C   uric acid
D   xanthine
E   calcium oxalate

38 A **True**   with proteinuria (Berger's disease)
    B **False**   this is characteristically painful
    C **True**
    D **False**   anaemia and bone pain
    E **True**

39 A **False**   parathyroid glands
    B **False**   atria of heart
    C **True**   1-alpha-hydroxylation in the kidneys
    D **True** ⎫ both have effects on autoregulation
    E **True** ⎭ of renal blood flow

40 A **True**
    B **True**
    C **False** ⎫ 90% of renal calculi are radio-opaque in contrast
    D **False** ⎭ to 10% of gallstones
    E **True**

Neurology

1 **In dystrophia myotonica**
   A the muscles are typically hypertrophied
   B weakness primarily affects the face, neck and forearms
   C the inheritance is usually autosomal recessive
   D fasciculation is an expected feature
   E ptosis is characteristic

2 **The Holmes–Adie syndrome is associated with**
   A loss of tendon reflexes
   B unilateral pupillary enlargement with delayed reaction to light
   C pupils which respond briskly to 1% tropicamide eye drops
   D a positive HIV status
   E a preponderance in females

3 **Wernicke's encephalopathy**
   A is due to thiamine deficiency
   B is associated with Korsakoff's psychosis
   C is a recognized complication of hyperemesis gravidarum
   D results from a lesion of the caudate nucleus
   E typically produces loss of pupillary reflexes

4 **The facial nerve**
   A traverses the parotid gland
   B supplies the orbicularis oculi muscle
   C enters the internal auditory meatus with the VIIIth nerve
   D supplies taste sensation to the posterior third of tongue
   E leaves the skull by the foramen ovale

5 **Pseudobulbar palsy is**
   A a feature of motor neurone disease
   B usually associated with an exaggerated jaw jerk
   C commonly due to bilateral internal capsule damage
   D characteristically associated with emotional lability
   E associated with absence of the palatal gag reflex

1	A	**False**	characterized by muscle wasting
	B	**True**	facial, sternomastoid, shoulder girdle and forearm muscles
	C	**False**	autosomal dominant inheritance
	D	**False**	
	E	**True**	
2	A	**True**	absence of tendon jerks especially ankle and knee jerks is characteristic
	B	**True**	pupil abnormality is unilateral in most patients (80%), moderately dilated pupil with sluggish or absent reaction to light
	C	**False**	pupils already dilated
	D	**False**	
	E	**True**	aetiology unknown
3	A	**True**	characterized by mental changes, ataxia, nystagmus and ophthalmoplegia
	B	**True**	in less severe and acute cases the mental changes are usually those of Korsakoff's psychosis
	C	**True**	associated conditions include alcoholism gastrointestinal disorders, hyperemesis gravidarum and malnourishment
	D	**False**	lesions occur in the hypothalamus and mammillary bodies particularly
	E	**False**	
4	A	**True**	
	B	**True**	it supplies all the muscles of facial expression
	C	**True**	
	D	**False**	nervus intermedius supplies taste to the anterior two-thirds of the tongue
	E	**False**	leaves the skull at the stylomastoid foramen
5	A	**True**	pseudobulbar palsy occurs with bilateral internal capsule damage whether vascular, demyelination or neoplastic infiltration; also in motor neurone disease
	B	**True**	
	C	**True**	
	D	**True**	the features also include dysarthria, dysphagia and increased jaw jerk
	E	**False**	preservation or exaggeration of the palatal gag reflex

6 **Absent knee jerks and extensor plantar responses are typical features of**
  A peroneal muscular atrophy
  B Friedreich's ataxia
  C vitamin B_{12} deficiency
  D tabes dorsalis
  E myotonia congenita

7 **Homonymous hemianopia is a recognized feature of**
  A chronic papilloedema
  B lesions of the optic tract
  C lesions in the posterior part of the parietal lobe
  D expanding pituitary neoplasms
  E thrombosis of the posterior cerebral artery

8 **When testing the cochlear component of the VIIIth cranial nerve**
  A nerve deafness results in louder air-conducted sound than bone-conducted sound
  B conduction deafness results in louder air-conducted sound than bone-conducted sound
  C in normal people, bone-conducted sound is louder than air-conducted sound
  D the base of the tuning fork is placed on the centre of the head in Rinne's test and on the mastoid in Weber's test
  E a tuning fork on the centre of the head is best perceived on the side of the middle ear disease

9 **In chronic subdural haematoma**
  A bleeding usually occurs from the middle meningeal artery
  B symptoms fluctuate from day to day
  C young adults are most frequently affected
  D a latent period is present before symptoms develop
  E a history of previous head injury is elicited in the majority of patients

10 **In general paralysis of the insane**
  A males are more often affected than females
  B delusions of grandeur occur in the majority of patients
  C cortical atrophy is a typical autopsy finding
  D presentation usually occurs within 5 years of the primary infection
  E transient hemiplegia is a recognized presentation

6 A **False** absent ankle jerks but normal or absent plantar
responses
  B **True**
  C **True**' lesions of the conus medullaris, spinal shock and
motor neurone disease also produce this picture
  D **False** syphilitic taboparesis (i.e. combined features of GPI
and tabes dorsalis—not tabes dorsalis alone)
  E **False**

---

7 A **False** scotomas not hemianopias
  B **True** lesions of the optic tract and posterior parietal lobe
  C **True**
  D **True** bitemporal hemianopia due to chiasmal pressure but
may involve one optic tract asymmetrically
  E **True**

---

8 A **True** as in normal people
  B **False** bone conduction is the greater
  C **False**
  D **False** the tuning fork is placed on the centre of the
forehead in Weber's test but close to the ear then on
the mastoid in Rinne's test
  E **True** extraneous background noise does not interfere with
perception on the side of conduction deafness

---

9 A **False** bleeding occurs from veins traversing the subdural
space
  B **True**
  C **False** elderly adults
  D **True**
  E **False** often minor unreported head injury

---

10 A **True**
   B **False** grandiose form is less common than simple
dementia
   C **True**
   D **False** usually develops 10–15 years after primary infection
   E **True** so-called 'congestive attacks'

11 **The posterior inferior cerebellar artery**
    A   is a branch of the basilar artery
    B   supplies the dorso-lateral portion of the medulla
    C   when occluded, damages the spinal tract and nucleus of the trigeminal nerve
    D   when occluded, results in unilateral pyramidal tract signs
    E   supplies the lower vestibular nuclei

12 **The following are typical fundoscopic features of papilloedema**
    A   prominence of lamina cribrosa
    B   pink disc with distinct margin
    C   dot haemorrhages
    D   engorged retinal veins
    E   looping of arterial vessels

13 **Recognized features of prefrontal lobe neoplasms include**
    A   homonymous hemianopia
    B   few localizing physical signs
    C   a grasp reflex in the contralateral hand
    D   intention tremor of the contralateral arm
    E   unilateral anosmia

14 **Recognized signs of cavernous sinus thrombosis include**
    A   unilateral exophthalmos
    B   papilloedema
    C   third nerve (oculomotor) palsy
    D   nerve deafness
    E   dysconjugate nystagmus

15 **Horner's syndrome (cervical sympathetic paralysis) results in**
    A   exophthalmos
    B   pupillary dilatation
    C   abolition of the cilio-spinal reflex on the ipsilateral side
    D   reduced sweating on ipsilateral side of face
    E   ptosis

11 A **False** a branch of the vertebral artery
    B **True**
    C **True** and damages the inferior cerebellar peduncle to produce ipsilateral cerebellar signs
    D **False** the pyramidal tract is supplied by the anterior spinal artery
    E **True** leading to nausea, vertigo and nystagmus if disordered

12 A **False** the following stages of papilloedema occur—engorgement of retinal veins, increased pinkness of optic disc, blurring of disc margins, filling of optic cup and haemorrhages around disc
    B **True**
    C **False** the micro-aneurysms of diabetic retinopathy
    D **True**
    E **False**

13 A **False** conjugate gaze palsies
    B **True** personality changes, incontinence of urine or faeces, adversive epileptic seizures, unilateral anosmia, contralateral grasp and groping reflexes and apraxia of gait; in dominant hemisphere lesions expressive dysphasia may occur
    C **True**
    D **False**
    E **True**

14 A **True**
    B **True**
    C **True** the III, IV and VI cranial nerves may be involved
    D **False** infection usually spreads from nasal sinuses and the VIIIth nerve is not involved
    E **False**

15 A **False** paralysis of the dilator of the iris with miosis, slight ptosis, enophthalmos and reduced sweating on the affected side of the face
    B **False**
    C **True** the pupil fails to dilate when the eye is shaded, in states of pain and emotional excitement and when the skin on the same side of the neck is scratched with a pin (cilio-spinal reflex)
    D **True**
    E **True**

16   **Clinical signs of injury to the posterior columns of the spinal cord include**
   A   astereognosis
   B   loss of vibration sense
   C   a positive Romberg's test
   D   dysdiadochokinesis
   E   loss of two-point discrimination

17   **Clinical signs of cerebellar dysfunction include**
   A   hypertonia
   B   dysmetria
   C   intention tremor
   D   pendular nystagmus
   E   scanning speech

18   **Findings consistent with syringomyelia include**
   A   early loss of position sense in the legs
   B   pain in the arms on coughing
   C   loss of sensation over the outer aspect of the face
   D   weakness of the intrinsic muscles of the hand
   E   preservation of the reflexes in the arms

19   **Division of the sciatic nerve produces**
   A   an absent ankle jerk
   B   global anaesthesia below the knee
   C   paralysis of adduction of the leg
   D   weakness of the quadriceps
   E   foot drop

20   **Recognized features of myasthenia gravis include**
   A   muscle spasm
   B   acetylcholine receptor antibodies
   C   reduction in the neuro-transmission at the motor end plate
   D   improvement with anticholinesterase drug therapy
   E   response to thymectomy in 90% of adults

16 A **True**
B **True** loss of vibration sense and joint position sense, hence sensory ataxia and a positive Romberg's test
C **True**
D **False** dysdiadochokinesis, rebound phenomenon, alternating movements are features of cerebellar disorders
E **True**

17 A **False** hypotonia, ataxia, dysmetria, dyssynergia, dysdiadochokinesis, rebound phenomenon, pendular tendon reflexes and dysarthria
B **True**
C **True**
D **False** nystagmus is jerking not pendular
E **True**

18 A **False** dissociated sensory loss with loss of pain and temperature sensation. Loss of position sense in the legs may occur but is a late sign
B **True**
C **True** involvement of the lower spinal tract of the V nerve impairs the sensation of the outer aspect of the face; the area of analgesia may converge upon the tip of the nose and the upper lip in the later stages
D **True**
E **False** the tendon reflexes in the arms are usually lost but are exaggerated in legs

19 A **True**
B **False** sensory loss over dorsum and sole of the foot (a substantial part of the sensory supply below the knee medially is supplied by the femoral nerve)
C **False** obturator nerve
D **False** femoral nerve
E **True** weakness occurs in dorsiflexion, plantar flexion, eversion and inversion of the foot and knee flexion

20 A **False** muscle weakness
B **True** receptor antibodies occur in approximately 90%
C **True**
D **True** responds to anticholinesterase agents although corticosteroids, azathioprine and thymectomy are also useful in management
E **False** children and young adults especially but is less predictable over the age of 40 years

21   **The ulnar nerve**
A   arises from lateral cord of brachial plexus
B   carries nerve fibres from C7 and C8
C   supplies only motor fibres to the hand
D   supplies adductor pollicis
E   supplies flexor carpi ulnaris

22   **Spastic paraplegia is a recognized feature of**
A   chronic lead poisoning
B   B$_{12}$ deficiency
C   cervical spondylosis
D   Hodgkin's disease
E   motor neurone disease

23   **A CSF protein concentration of greater than 3 g/l is an expected finding in**
A   multiple sclerosis
B   epidural abscess
C   acoustic neuroma
D   motor neurone disease
E   Guillain–Barré syndrome

24   **In Huntington's disease**
A   the condition is inherited as an autosomal dominant trait
B   spastic paraplegia is a recognized late feature
C   optic atrophy occurs early in the disease
D   the disease usually appears in the second and third decades
E   early treatment can prevent the development of dementia

25   **In multiple sclerosis**
A   diplopia without objective ocular palsy is a recognized feature
B   presentation with widespread paraesthesia carries a poor prognosis
C   abdominal reflexes are absent in the majority of patients
D   there is an association with histocompatibility antigens HLA A3 and DR2
E   onset after the age of 60 years is a characteristic feature

21   A   **False**   arises from the medial cord of the brachial plexus
     B   **False**   spinal nerves C8 and T1
     C   **False**   sensory supply is to the fifth and lateral half of the fourth finger. Motor supply is to flexor carpi ulnaris, ulnar half of flexor digitorum profundus, palmaris brevis, muscles of the hypothenar eminence, the two medial lumbricals, the palmar and dorsal interossei, adductor pollicis and flexor pollicis brevis
     D   **True**
     E   **True**

22   A   **False**   motor polyneuropathy
     B   **True**   vitamin B_{12} deficiency, cervical myelopathy, motor neurone disease, sagittal sinus thrombosis, parasagittal meningioma, multiple sclerosis and epidural tumour are the main differential diagnoses
     C   **True**
     D   **True**
     E   **True**

23   A   **False**   CSF total protein is normal (0.3 to 0.6 g/l) but the gamma globulin fraction is elevated (> 12% of total).
     B   **True**   Acoustic neuroma, Guillain–Barré syndrome and Froin's syndrome (spinal block due to tumour or epidural abscess) are accompanied by a marked rise in CSF protein
     C   **True**
     D   **False**
     E   **True**

24   A   **True**
     B   **False**   spastic paraplegia and optic atrophy do not occur
     C   **False**
     D   **False**   personality change, dementia and chorea appear in the fourth decade or later
     E   **False**   no treatment is known to influence the disease

25   A   **True**   often a subtle internuclear ophthalmoplegia
     B   **False**   sensory forms of the condition are relatively benign
     C   **True**   abdominal reflexes are lost in two-thirds of cases
     D   **True**
     E   **False**   presentation is uncommon after 50 years and rare after 60

26   **Miotic pupils are a typical feature of**
   A   tabes dorsalis
   B   retro-bulbar neuritis
   C   Holmes–Adie syndrome
   D   tricyclic antidepressant poisoning
   E   oculomotor nerve palsy

27   **Characteristic features of temporal lobe neoplasms include**
   A   motor dysphasia
   B   apraxia
   C   complex partial seizures
   D   a positive grasp reflex
   E   homonymous visual field defects

28   **Signs indicating a lower motor neurone lesion include**
   A   fasciculation
   B   clonus
   C   hypotonicity
   D   wasting
   E   extensor plantar response

29   **Facial paralysis is an expected finding in**
   A   acoustic neuroma
   B   pontine neoplasm
   C   thrombosis of the medial striate branches of the middle
       cerebral artery
   D   parotid neoplasm
   E   posterior inferior cerebellar artery thrombosis

30   **In the innervation of the lower limb**
   A   the T12 root supplies the sensation over the anterior thigh
   B   the L5 root supplies the sensation over the 5th toe
   C   the common peroneal nerve supplies the dorsi-flexors of the
       toes
   D   the hip flexors are innervated by the roots L2–L3
   E   the S1–S2 roots supply sensation to the perineum

31   **Recognized causes of epileptic fits include**
   A   hypoglycaemia
   B   multiple sclerosis
   C   diazepam withdrawal
   D   general paralysis of the insane
   E   mefenamic acid overdosage

26 A **True**   Argyll Robertson pupils
    B **False**
    C **False** retrobulbar neuritis, Holmes–Adie syndrome, IIIrd
                  nerve palsy and tricyclic overdosage all lead to
                  mydriasis
    D **False**
    E **False**

27 A **False** nominal or receptive (sensory) dysphasia
    B **False** a feature of parietal lobe lesions
    C **True**
    D **False** a sign of a frontal lobe lesion
    E **True**   especially upper quadrantinopia

28 A **True**   muscle wasting, fasciculation, hypotonia and loss of
                  tendon reflexes
    B **False** clonus and extensor plantar responses are features
                  of upper motor neurone lesions
    C **True**
    D **True**
    E **False**

29 A **True**   also pontine and posterior fossa neoplasms
    B **True**
    C **True**   an upper motor neurone facial palsy
    D **True**   courses through the parotid
    E **False** a medullary infarct below the facial nerve nuclei

30 A **False** sensation superior to the inguinal ligament
    B **False** sensation over the large toe (1st), 2nd and 3rd. S1
                  supplies the 4th and 5th toes
    C **True**   the common peroneal supplies the dorsi-flexors and
                  evertors of the ankle
    D **True**
    E **False** S2,3,4 supply the perineum

31 A **True**   important to remember
    B **True**   uncommon except in advanced disease
    C **True**
    D **True**   epilepsy occurs in 50% of patients
    E **True**   characteristic

32 Jerking nystagmus is a recognized feature of

A albinism
B multiple sclerosis
C Friedreich's ataxia
D tabes dorsalis
E vestibular neuronitis

33 In a patient with the clinical features suggesting raised intracranial pressure

A lumbar puncture should be performed immediately to exclude meningitis
B headache is most often bilateral and worse in the morning
C sixth (abducens) cranial nerve paresis is common
D loss of visual acuity is an early symptom
E erosion of the clinoids of the dorsum sellae on skull X-rays suggest long-standing intracranial disease

34 Neurological manifestations of the acquired immunodeficiency syndrome include

A painful sensorimotor polyneuropathy
B subacute encephalitis
C cerebral atrophy
D proximal myopathy
E cerebral lymphoma

35 Characteristic features of Guillain–Barré syndrome include

A bladder dysfunction
B normal CSF protein
C satisfactory response to oral prednisolone
D loss of limb reflexes
E complete recovery within 6 months

36 Peripheral neuropathy is a common complication of

A pellagra
B infectious mononucleosis
C myeloma
D Cushing's syndrome
E Behçet's disease

32 A **False** pendular nystagmus
    B **True**   occurs with labyrinthine and cerebellar disorders
                  including Ménière's disease, disseminated sclerosis,
                  Friedreich's ataxia and vestibular neuronitis
    C **True**
    D **False** unless associated with GPI (taboparesis)
    E **True**

33 A **False** lumbar puncture should be deferred until CT
                  scanning is undertaken; if necessary, antibiotics can
                  be given pending the result
    B **True**   may waken the patient from sleep
    C **True**   'false localizing' sign
    D **False** loss of visual acuity occurs late in papilloedema
    E **True**

34 A **True**   one of the commoner manifestations
    B **True**   affects most patients who survive long enough
    C **True**   causes a dementia-like syndrome
    D **True**   usually due to zidovudine treatment
    E **True**   AIDS-related malignancy

35 A **False** if present, raises the suspicion of spinal cord
                  compression
    B **False** CSF protein is characteristically high and may lead to
                  papilloedema
    C **False** rarely effective
    D **True**
    E **True**

36 A **True**
    B **False** rare manifestation
    C **True**   can improve with treatment if not due to amyloidosis
    D **False** proximal myopathy is common
    E **False** vasculitis and demyelination occurs in brain stem,
                  cerebellum and long tracts

37   **Dementia is a characteristic feature of**
  A   Parkinson's disease
  B   normal pressure hydrocephalus
  C   Shy–Drager syndrome
  D   Wilson's disease
  E   metachromatic leucodystrophy

38   **Involuntary movement disorders are a typical feature of**
  A   thyrotoxicosis
  B   hypokalaemic periodic paralysis
  C   dystrophia myotonica
  D   encephalitis lethargica
  E   tardive dyskinesia

39   **A 54-year-old man presents with his first generalized tonic–clonic seizure resulting in left arm and left leg weakness which resolves after 72 hours. Useful initial investigations include**
  A   examination of cerebro-spinal fluid
  B   somato-sensory evoked potentials (SSEP)
  C   contrast-enhanced CT scanning of brain
  D   electro-encephalogram
  E   digital subtraction angiography

40   **Preferred single-drug therapy of generalized epilepsy includes**
  A   selegiline
  B   lamotrigine
  C   clonazepam
  D   ethosuximide
  E   sodium valproate

37 A **False**   parkinsonism often accompanies severe dementia
    B **True**   with urinary incontinence and ataxic gait
    C **False**   a progressive autonomic failure when degenerative
                   changes affect basal ganglia, cerebellum, brain stem
                   and intermediolateral column of spinal cord
    D **True**   if advanced and untreated
    E **True**

38 A **False**   exaggerated physiological tremor
    B **False**   episodes of weakness provoked by exercise or meals
    C **False**
    D **True**   post-encephalitic parkinsonism
    E **True**   a serious side-effect of continuous neuroleptic
                   therapy

39 A **False**   potentially hazardous and unhelpful at this stage in
                   the investigation
    B **False**   useful in sensory pathway lesions especially in
                   spinal roots, spinal and brachial plexus
    C **True**   mandatory since neoplasm causing Todd's paresis is
                   a possible diagnosis
    D **False**   likely to be non-specifically abnormal
    E **False**

40 A **False**   useful in Parkinson's disease
    B **True**   especially if resistant to first-line drugs
    C **True**   especially myoclonus and absences
    D **True**   useful in absence seizures
    E **True**   useful in partial and generalized epilepsies

Respiratory medicine

1 In the normal pulmonary circulation
   A pulmonary veins drain blood from both pulmonary and bronchial arteries
   B the azygous vein drains into the left atrium directly
   C the pulmonary artery supplies the capillary bed in the bronchial walls
   D the pulmonary arterioles dilate in response to hypoxia
   E in the erect position the upper zones are less well perfused than the mid or lower zones

2 Typical manifestations of ventilatory failure include
   A drowsiness
   B cold extremities
   C papilloedema
   D flapping tremor
   E muscle twitching

3 Transfer factor (T_{CO}), as measured using the single breath method, is
   A greater in childhood than in adulthood
   B higher in males than in females
   C reduced by exercise
   D increased in polycythaemia
   E reduced in chronic pulmonary sarcoidosis

4 Alveolar hypoventilation is an expected complication of
   A gross obesity
   B hysteria
   C myasthenia gravis
   D kyphoscoliosis
   E pulmonary oedema

5 In a subject breathing air at sea level an arterial PaO_2 of 7.5 kPa and arterial $PaCO_2$ of 4.5 kPa are typical of
   A farmer's lung
   B morphine overdosage
   C lobar pneumonia
   D lymphangitis carcinomatosis
   E deep sleep

1   A   **True**
     B   **False**   the azygous vein drains into the superior vena cava
     C   **False**   pulmonary arteries supply alveolar capillaries and
                         bronchial arteries supply the bronchial and
                         bronchiolar walls
     D   **False**   hypoxia and acidosis cause pulmonary arterial
                         constriction
     E   **True**   gravity influences blood flow within the lung

2   A   **True**   ventilatory failure causes drowsiness, headaches,
                         warm extremities, a flapping tremor, muscle
                         twitching, sweating and tachycardia
     B   **False**
     C   **True**
     D   **True**
     E   **True**

3   A   **True**   the T_{CO} is affected by the haemoglobin
                         concentration, ventilation-perfusion matching, the
                         alveolar surface area and the characteristics of the
                         alveolar membrane
     B   **True**
     C   **False**   increased by exercise and increased cardiac output
     D   **True** T_{CO} is reduced in anaemia
     E   **True**

4   A   **True**   reduced alveolar ventilation may be due to uneven
                         distribution of inspired air, insensitivity of the
                         respiratory centre to $PaCO_2$ or reduced chest wall
                         expansion
     B   **False**
     C   **True**
     D   **True**
     E   **False**   hysteria and pulmonary oedema are usually
                         associated with hyperventilation

5   A   **True**   type 1 respiratory failure is associated with
                         interstitial lung disease and loss of effective alveolar
                         surface area
     B   **False** $PaCO_2$ rises due to respiratory depression
     C   **True**
     D   **True**
     E   **False**

6   Characteristic changes in lung function in emphysema include
A   normal functional residual capacity (FRC)
B   reduced FEV_1
C   normal FEV_1/FVC ratio
D   raised RV/TLC ratio
E   reduced T_{CO}

7   In the normal lung
A   the right main bronchus is more vertical than the left
B   the right upper lobe has four segmental bronchi
C   the bronchioli contain no cartilage or mucous glands
D   the left lower lobe has five segmental bronchi
E   an azygous lobe is present in 5% of left lungs

8   In the oxygen dissociation curve
A   the shape and position of the curve are affected by body temperature
B   acidosis shifts the curve to the left
C   massive blood transfusion shifts the curve to the right
D   the curve is abnormal in haemoglobin Chesapeake
E   the curve relates the percentage oxygen saturation to the alveolar arterial oxygen tension gradient

9   Products of arachidonic acid metabolism include
A   thromboxane A_2
B   prostacyclin
C   histamine
D   leukotriene B_4
E   bradykinin

10   A lateral chest X-ray which reveals a mass posteriorly overlying the spine suggests the possibility of a
A   thymoma
B   tuberculous abscess
C   pericardial cyst
D   bronchogenic cyst
E   neuroblastoma

6 A **False** emphysema is characterized by an obstructive defect with low FEV_1/FVC ratio and raised FRC and RV/TLC ratio
   B **True**
   C **False**
   D **True**
   E **True** the alveolar surface area and therefore the T_{CO} are reduced

7 A **True** the right main bronchus is shorter and more vertical than the left
   B **False** the right upper lobe contains three segments, the left lower four
   C **True**
   D **False**
   E **False** azygous lobes occur only on the right

8 A **True**
   B **False** acidosis moves the curve to the right, alkalosis to the left
   C **False** transfused blood contains less 2,3-diphosphoglycerate, a haemoglobin ligand, and can shift the curve to the left
   D **True** abnormal haemoglobins transfer less oxygen
   E **False**

9 A **True** cyclo-oxygenase converts arachidonic acid to prostacyclin and prostaglandins, while 5-lipoxygenase stimulates leukotriene production
   B **True**
   C **False** histamine and bradykinin are preformed within the mast cell
   D **True**
   E **False**

10 A **False** the thymus lies anteriorly
   B **True** TB abscesses may arise from the vertebrae
   C **False** pericardial cysts occur at the anterior cardiophrenic angle
   D **False** bronchogenic cysts occur in the anterior and superior mediastinum
   E **True**

11   Miliary calcification of the lungs is a recognized feature of
   A   histoplasmosis
   B   asbestosis
   C   chickenpox
   D   sarcoidosis
   E   silicosis

12   The phrenic nerve
   A   is derived from C6 and C7 spinal roots
   B   contains only motor fibres
   C   on the left, lies anterior to the aortic arch
   D   when paralysed causes the affected hemidiaphragm to descend on sniffing
   E   can be stimulated by skin electrodes on the neck

13   During a moderately severe attack of acute asthma, the typical alterations in pulmonary function include
   A   decreased arterial PaO_2
   B   increased arterial $PaCO_2$
   C   decreased functional residual capacity (FRC)
   D   raised serum bicarbonate concentration
   E   decreased peak expiratory flow rate (PEFR)

14   Characteristic findings in cor pulmonale due to chronic obstructive airways disease include
   A   ascites
   B   tricuspid incompetence
   C   left bundle branch block on ECG
   D   pallor
   E   enlargement of hilar shadows on chest X-ray

15   Factors implicated in the aetiology of chronic bronchitis and emphysema include
   A   cigarette smoking
   B   recurrent chest infections
   C   whooping cough pneumonia in childhood
   D   atmospheric pollution with sulphur dioxide
   E   alpha$_1$-antitrypsin deficiency

11	A	**True**	fine nodular calcification on chest X-ray may occur following chickenpox and histoplasmosis
	B	**False**	diffuse fibrosis and pleural plaques
	C	**True**	
	D	**False**	bilateral hilar lymphadenopathy, pulmonary infiltrates and even miliary mottling but not calcification
	E	**False**	'egg-shell' calcification of enlarged hilar lymph nodes

12	A	**False**	the phrenic nerve is derived from C3–5; mainly C4
	B	**False**	some afferent fibres, hence referred diaphragmatic pain
	C	**True**	
	D	**False**	when paralysed the hemidiaphragm is elevated and moves paradoxically during respiration
	E	**True**	

13	A	**True**	FEV_1 and PEFR fall due to bronchospasm and FRC rises due to 'air trapping'. Arterial PaO_2 is reduced but $PaCO_2$ remains low or normal unless extremely severe
	B	**False**	
	C	**False**	
	D	**False**	metabolic acidosis may occur in children with acute asthma
	E	**True**	

14	A	**True**	peripheral oedema, ascites and a raised JVP are typical and in the later stages tricuspid incompetence frequently occurs
	B	**True**	
	C	**False**	RBBB may be seen on ECG
	D	**False**	plethora and polycythaemia are often found
	E	**True**	secondary to pulmonary arterial hypertension

15	A	**True**	cigarette smoking and atmospheric pollution, particularly SO_2, are associated with chronic bronchitis and emphysema
	B	**False**	
	C	**False**	bronchiectasis
	D	**True**	
	E	**False**	alpha$_1$-antitrypsin deficiency causes panacinar emphysema but not bronchitis

16   **An adolescent female with a history of chronic respiratory disease is found to have bronchiectasis. The following would be helpful in establishing the aetiology**
   A   a long-standing history of diarrhoea with pale stools
   B   a positive precipitin reaction to *Aspergillus fumigatus*
   C   a history of a severe attack of whooping cough
   D   dextrocardia
   E   calcified bronchopulmonary lymph nodes on X-ray

17   **Radical surgical treatment for bronchial carcinoma is contraindicated by**
   A   peripheral neuropathy
   B   grossly widened carina on bronchoscopy
   C   hoarseness with a bovine cough
   D   FEV 0.8 litre
   E   raised right hemidiaphragm which descends on sniffing

18   **The post-operative survival rate in lung cancer is reduced if**
   A   the patient is over 60 years old
   B   the tumour is of small-cell type
   C   there has been weight loss of over 10 lb approximately
   D   the tumour affects the left lung
   E   pneumonectomy is undertaken

19   **Recognized findings in a Pancoast tumour include**
   A   severe shoulder pain
   B   contralateral ptosis
   C   paralysis of the muscles in the forearm
   D   pain in the arm radiating to the 4th and 5th fingers
   E   gangrene of the fingers of the same side

20   **Inhaled materials predisposing to lung cancer include**
   A   sandstone
   B   chromates
   C   beryllium
   D   carbonyl nickel
   E   chloromethyl ether

16   A   **True**   cystic fibrosis may be associated with pancreatic
                     steatorrhoea
     B   **False**   bronchiectasis can occur after allergic
                     bronchopulmonary aspergillosis, a positive precipitin
                     reaction is of no diagnostic help however
     C   **True**   bronchiectasis may occur after measles, whooping
                     cough or tuberculosis
     D   **True**   Kartagener's syndrome with absent frontal sinuses,
                     dextrocardia and bronchiectasis
     E   **True**   TB

17   A   **False**   non-metastatic complication
     B   **True**   mediastinal glands are involved
     C   **True**   involvement of recurrent laryngeal nerve
     D   **True**   poor lung function associated with poor outcome
     E   **False**   not a phrenic nerve palsy!

18   A   **True**   favourable prognostic factors in the post-operative
                     survival of lung cancer include age under 60,
                     operation on the right side (right lung is bigger) and
                     a lobectomy rather than pneumonectomy
     B   **True**   small-cell carcinomas metastasize early
     C   **True**   metastatic disease is more likely
     D   **True**
     E   **True**

19   A   **True**   an apical lung tumour may erode the first rib to
                     produce severe shoulder pain and involve the
                     sympathetic nerves to produce an ipsilateral
                     Horner's syndrome
     B   **False**
     C   **True**   damaged C8 and T1 nerve roots cause pain in 4th
                     and 5th digits and paralysis of forearm and hand
     D   **True**
     E   **False**   the arterial circulation is not compromised

20   A   **False**   silicosis with pulmonary infiltrates
     B   **True**   chrome ore and asbestos predispose to carcinoma
     C   **False**   beryllium causes granulomata
     D   **True**   squamous-cell carcinoma
     E   **True**   small-cell carcinoma

21   **Associations with carcinoma of the bronchus include**
A   alopecia totalis
B   psoriasis
C   hypokalaemic alkalosis
D   sensory neuropathy
E   arthropathy

22   **In BCG vaccination**
A   an attenuated live strain of *Mycobacterium bovis* is used
B   protective efficacy rates are similar world-wide
C   protection against leprosy is conferred
D   mild regional adenitis commonly occurs afterwards
E   in the United Kingdom, it is recommended for all tuberculin-negative children at 2 years of age

23   **Toxic effects of rifampicin include**
A   optic neuropathy
B   pyridoxine deficiency
C   deranged liver function tests
D   decreased effectiveness of warfarin therapy
E   haemolytic anaemia

24   **Recognized findings in acute miliary tuberculosis include**
A   normal chest X-ray
B   negative tuberculin test
C   aplastic anaemia
D   occurrence in individuals who have previously been successfully vaccinated with BCG
E   haemoptysis

25   **Characteristic features of Legionnaire's disease include**
A   confusion
B   lymphocytosis
C   hypophosphataemia
D   hypernatraemia
E   diarrhoea

21 A **False**
    B **False**
    C **True**   ectopic ACTH secretion produces hypokalaemic alkalosis
    D **True**   carcinomatous neuropathy
    E **True**   hypertrophic osteoarthropathy is usually due to squamous carcinoma not small-cell carcinoma

22 A **True**
    B **False**   variable protection rates of 0–84% but good protection against human and bovine TB and leprosy
    C **True**
    D **True**   ulceration of the wound and regional adenitis
    E **False**   it is offered mainly to subjects in high-risk groups

23 A **False**   ethambutol produces optic neuropathy; isoniazid produces peripheral neuropathy due to pyridoxine deficiency
    B **False**
    C **True**
    D **True**   the metabolism of corticosteroids, oral contraceptives, warfarin and sulphonylureas is increased
    E **True**

24 A **True**   tubercles may be too small to be seen on X-ray
    B **True**
    C **True**   splenomegaly and aplastic anaemia disappear with treatment
    D **False**   miliary TB and TB meningitis do not occur in patients who have had successful BCG vaccination
    E **False**   post-primary cavitating pulmonary TB

25 A **True**   pneumonia with systemic symptoms including confusion, arthralgia, vomiting and diarrhoea
    B **False**   moderate leucocytosis with relative lymphopenia is typical
    C **True**   typical of severe sepsis
    D **False**   hyponatraemia and hypophosphataemia occur in about 50% of cases
    E **True**

26   Characteristic radiological findings in cryptogenic fibrosing alveolitis include
- **A** hyperinflation
- **B** a honeycomb pattern
- **C** pleural plaques
- **D** bilateral involvement
- **E** hilar lymphadenopathy

27   A woman aged 30 years has previously suffered from red, tender nodules over her shins and now presents with a pyrexial illness. Chest X-ray shows bilateral hilar enlargement and the tuberculin test is negative. Additional expected findings include
- **A** lacrimal gland enlargement
- **B** facial palsy
- **C** hypercalciuria
- **D** pleural effusion
- **E** elevated serum angiotensin-converting enzyme

28   Characteristic features of farmer's lung include
- **A** immediate onset after exposure to mouldy hay
- **B** severe wheezing and lacrimation
- **C** fever
- **D** precipitin to *Micropolyspora faeni* in the serum
- **E** a restrictive pattern on spirometry

29   Features of cryptogenic fibrosing alveolitis include
- **A** exertional breathlessness
- **B** hypertrophic pulmonary osteoarthropathy
- **C** dysphagia
- **D** fine basal crepitations which clear on coughing
- **E** non-productive cough

30   The effects of positive end-expiratory pressure (PEEP) in the treatment of the adult respiratory distress syndrome (ARDS) include
- **A** a fall in functional residual capacity (FRC)
- **B** an increased oxygen saturation in the arteries
- **C** the prevention or delay of oxygen-induced lung damage
- **D** a rise in cardiac output
- **E** the risk of pulmonary barotrauma

31   Recognized associations with pneumothorax include
- **A** exposure to aluminium dust
- **B** acute pulmonary oedema
- **C** Ehlers–Danlos syndrome
- **D** pulmonary tuberculosis
- **E** pleural mesothelioma

26 A **False**   bilateral shrunken lung fields with a ground glass, miliary or honeycomb pattern

     B **True**

     C **False**

     D **True**

     E **False**

---

27 A **True**   typical picture of sarcoidosis. Cranial nerve palsies, hypercalcaemia, hypercalciuria and lacrimal gland enlargement are recognized associations

     B **True**

     C **True**

     D **False**   pleural effusions in sarcoid are rare

     E **True**   occurs in 60% with active disease

---

28 A **False**   an extrinsic allergic alveolitis

     B **False**

     C **True**   fever, cough and breathlessness without wheeze occur 6 hours after exposure

     D **True**

     E **True**

---

29 A **True**   progressive breathlessness with type 1 respiratory failure

     B **True**   finger clubbing is usually obvious

     C **False**

     D **False**   crackles do not clear on coughing

     E **True**   characteristic and intractable

---

30 A **False**   raises FRC to improve oxygen saturation

     B **True**

     C **True**   allows ventilation with lower concentrations of oxygen to minimize oxygen-induced damage

     D **False**   cardiac output falls

     E **True**

---

31 A **True**   occurs in many occupational lung diseases, e.g. aluminium exposure, silicosis, berylliosis, in diseases with abnormal connective tissue such as Ehlers–Danlos with subpleural cysts, and in cavitating pulmonary tuberculosis

     B **False**

     C **True**

     D **True**

     E **False**

32   **Recognized pulmonary manifestations of untreated rheumatoid arthritis include**
  A   bronchiolitis obliterans
  B   pulmonary eosinophilia
  C   pulmonary infarction
  D   rheumatoid nodules
  E   pleural effusions

33   **Features of primary pulmonary hypertension include**
  A   angina pectoris
  B   raised $PaCO_2$
  C   early diastolic murmur which is louder on expiration
  D   giant 'a' wave in the jugular venous pulse
  E   inverted P waves on ECG

34   **Precipitating antibodies are present in**
  A   bird fancier's lung
  B   bagassosis
  C   idiopathic pulmonary haemosiderosis
  D   fibrosing alveolitis
  E   pulmonary mycetoma

35   **Periodic respiration is a recognized feature of**
  A   pulmonary infarction
  B   head injury
  C   meningitis
  D   diabetic ketoacidosis
  E   left ventricular failure

36   **Characteristic findings on examination of pleural fluid include**
  A   a low glucose concentration in rheumatoid arthritis
  B   a protein concentration of 5 g/l in mesothelioma
  C   numerous polymorphs in tuberculosis
  D   numerous eosinophils and RBCs in pulmonary infarction
  E   raised amylase in effusion following pancreatitis

37   **Features of idiopathic pulmonary haemosiderosis include**
  A   recurrent haemoptysis
  B   onset over the age of 40 years
  C   hypochromic anaemia
  D   pulmonary fibrosis
  E   good response to desferrioxamine

32   A   **True**   pleural effusions, fibrosing alveolitis, nodules,
                      bronchiolitis obliterans and apical fibrosis
     B   **False**
     C   **False**   pulmonary infarction is curiously rare
     D   **True**
     E   **True**   especially common in men

33   A   **True**   severe dyspnoea, syncopal attacks and angina
     B   **False**   hyperventilation and low $PaCO_2$
     C   **False**   the early diastolic murmur of Graham–Steell fades
                      on expiration
     D   **True**   right atrial hypertrophy with P pulmonale on ECG
     E   **False**

34   A   **True**   precipitating antibodies against avian antigen and
                      sugar cane are found in bird fancier's lung and
                      bagassosis respectively
     B   **True**
     C   **False**
     D   **False**   in fibrosing alveolitis rheumatoid factor and ANF
                      may be found in 30%
     E   **True**   most aspergillomas have positive serum precipitins

35   A   **False**   tachypnoea or hyperpnoea
     B   **True**   periodic respiration (variable periods of apnoea) is
                      associated with raised intracranial pressure, brain
                      stem vascular disease and circulatory failure
     C   **True**
     D   **False**   hyperpnoea
     E   **True**

36   A   **True**
     B   **False**   malignant pleural effusions are usually exudates, i.e.
                      protein greater than 30 g/l
     C   **False**   lymphocytosis is typical in tuberculous effusions
     D   **True**
     E⋅ **True**

37   A   **True**   a rare disease affecting children and young adults,
                      characterized by recurrent haemoptysis, pulmonary
                      X-ray shadowing and hypochromic anaemia
     B   **False**
     C   **True**
     D   **True**   mediastinal lymphadenopathy can also occur
     E   **False**   blood transfusion when necessary is the only
                      supportive treatment

38 Causes of occupational asthma include
A toluene di-isocyanate
B platinum salts
C formalin
D mouldy cork dust
E flour dust

39 Cavitating pulmonary lesions are characteristic of
A systemic lupus erythematosus
B squamous-cell carcinoma
C Wegener's granulomatosis
D progressive massive fibrosis
E adult respiratory distress syndrome

40 Hypertrophic pulmonary osteo-arthropathy
A occurs in association with gynaecomastia
B is associated with pleural fibromas
C can involve the small joints of the spine
D is usually associated with small-cell carcinoma of the bronchus
E regresses following vagotomy or tumour resection

38 A **True**
    B **True**   occupational asthma can be caused by many agents
                   including isocyanates, platinum salts, proteolytic
                   enzymes, soldering flux and flour dust (baker's
                   asthma)
    C **True**
    D **False**   suberosis is an allergic alveolitis
    E **True**

39 A **False**   SLE produces pleural effusions and diffuse fibrotic
                   shadowing
    B **True**
    C **True**
    D **True**   also TB and staphylococcal bronchopneumonia
    E **False**   ARDS causes extensive 'fluffy' shadowing

40 A **True**   usually associated with bronchogenic carcinoma
                   (most often with squamous-cell and not small-cell)
                   and pleural tumours
    B **True**
    C **False**   joint stiffness and pain in the long bones (wrists,
                   ankles and knees)
    D **False**
    E **True**

Rheumatology

1 **The diagnosis of prolapsed intervertebral disc is unlikely if**
A there is evidence of multiple nerve root compression
B root involvement is bilateral and symmetrical
C sphincter involvement is apparent
D back pain and tenderness are diffuse
E back pain is unremitting and worse on resting

2 **Contraindications to cervical manipulation for neck pain include**
A sensory loss or paraesthesiae in the upper limbs
B pyramidal tract signs in the lower limbs
C minor radiological changes of cervical spondylosis
D pain radiating over the occiput
E cervical subluxation on X-ray

3 **Arthoscopy is indicated in the diagnosis of**
A a haemophilic joint
B an unexplained synovitis
C suspected tuberculous arthritis
D internal derangements of the knee
E loose bodies in the knee

4 **In carpal tunnel syndrome**
A pain is confined to the hand and forearm
B wasting of the hypothenar muscles is characteristic
C pregnancy aggravates the condition
D the radial pulse is reduced
E pain may be felt in the 5th finger

5 **Polyarthritis is a feature of**
A Sjögren's disease
B ulcerative colitis
C dermatomyositis
D polymyalgia rheumatica
E thalassaemia

1	A	**True**	indicates a more diffuse lesion
	B	**True**	disc protrusion usually occurs postero-laterally and therefore affects one side
	C	**False**	may result from a cauda equina compression
	D	**True**	acute prolapsed intervertebral disc causes local tenderness and pain in the root distribution
	E	**True**	systemic diseases, e.g. sacro-iliitis and malignancy should be suspected

2	A	**True**	indicate neurological compression; manipulation may cause permanent neurological damage
	B	**True**	
	C	**False**	X-ray to exclude spinal instability
	D	**False**	
	E	**True**	rare in cervical spondylosis but common in rheumatoid arthritis

3	A	**False**	needle aspiration only if infection requires exclusion
	B	**True**	pathology of atypical synovitis can be difficult to diagnose
	C	**False**	needle aspiration alone
	D	**True**	
	E	**True**	

4	A	**False**	pain may be felt in the upper arm, shoulder or root of neck
	B	**False**	hypothenar muscles are innervated by the ulnar nerve; the median nerve innervates the thenar muscles
	C	**True**	fluid retention
	D	**False**	radial artery lies superficial to the transverse carpal ligament
	E	**True**	innervation by the median nerve via nerve fibres from the ulnar nerve may supply the 5th finger

5	A	**True**	association of dry mouth and eyes and systemic connective tissue disorder (usually rheumatoid arthritis)
	B	**True**	characteristically associated with a lower limb arthritis
	C	**True**	heliotrope discoloration over elbows, knees and knuckles; causes contractures secondary to muscle involvement. Rarely, erosive arthritis may affect peripheral and spinal joints
	D	**True**	can affect the knees and sternoclavicular joints
	E	**False**	

6   Recognized complications of rheumatoid disease include
A   obliterative bronchiolitis
B   aortic valvulitis
C   mononeuritis multiplex
D   onycholysis
E   fibrosing alveolitis

7   In rheumatoid arthritis
A   the small joints of the feet are often involved
B   rheumatoid nodules are invariably associated with a strongly positive rheumatoid factor
C   palpable splenomegaly occurs in 25% of patients
D   rheumatoid vasculitis is characteristically associated with a peripheral neuropathy
E   the disease does not involve the intervertebral discs

8   Presenting features of rheumatoid arthritis indicating a poor prognosis include
A   rheumatoid factor in high titre
B   acute onset
C   rheumatoid nodules
D   erosive joint changes
E   onset after the age of 40 years

9   Rheumatoid factor
A   is present in infective endocarditis
B   is present in low titre in 4 to 5% of the general population
C   is an antibody against an abnormal immunoglobulin
D   when present early in the disease, is associated with an increased likelihood of progressive rheumatoid disease
E   is invariably present in severe rheumatoid diseases

10   In normal synovial fluid
A   the fluid is clear and colourless
B   the white cell count is usually 5–10 $\times$ 10^9 cells per litre
C   the viscosity is low
D   the fibrin content is high
E   the predominant white cell is the lymphocyte

11   Indications for treatment with gold or penicillamine include
A   recurrent palindromic rheumatism
B   progressive ankylosing spondylitis
C   progressive psoriatic arthritis
D   severe erosive juvenile arthritis
E   severe extra-articular manifestation of rheumatoid arthritis

6	A	**True**	may be associated with penicillamine therapy
	B	**True**	granulomatous inflammation damages the valve
	C	**True**	vasculitis
	D	**False**	seronegative arthropathy, especially Reiter's or psoriasis
	E	**True**	rheumatoid factor present in 30%

7	A	**True**	MTP and MCP joints are most often involved at onset
	B	**True**	immune complex deposition causing connective tissue damage
	C	**False**	usually only palpable in Felty's syndrome
	D	**True**	vasculitis involves the vasa nervora
	E	**False**	rheumatoid discitis

8	A	**True**	high titres of rheumatoid factor indicate a greater activation of the immune system
	B	**False**	even if severe at onset there may be no recurrence
	C	**True**	immune complexes and connective tissue damage are more often associated with chronic disease
	D	**True**	early erosions indicate active, progressive disease
	E	**False**	

9	A	**True**	rheumatoid factor is a mixture of IgM antibodies cross-reacting with normal IgG. In SBE, bacteria may stimulate the production of cross-reactive IgM
	B	**True**	increases with age
	C	**False**	antibody against normal IgG
	D	**True**	
	E	**False**	30% of patients with rheumatoid arthritis are seronegative

10	A	**True**	
	B	**False**	$0.2–1 \times 10^9$ per litre
	C	**False**	high viscosity
	D	**False**	fibrin indicates inflammation
	E	**True**	

11	A	**True**	in palindromic rheumatism, attacks are self-limiting and recurrent; these treatments may prevent relapse
	B	**False**	
	C	**True**	
	D	**True**	
	E	**True**	

12   Clinical features of psoriatic arthritis include
  A   distal interphalangeal joint involvement
  B   symmetrical joint involvement
  C   arthritis mutilans
  D   sacro-iliitis
  E   temporomandibular joint involvement

13   HLA B27 antigen is associated with arthritis in
  A   Forrestier's disease
  B   Behçet's disease
  C   yersiniosis
  D   shigellosis
  E   Still's disease

14   Recognized features of Reiter's syndrome include
  A   equal sex incidence
  B   keratoderma blenorrhagica
  C   urethritis in both enterically and sexually acquired disease
  D   painless buccal ulceration
  E   sacro-iliitis

15   Ankylosing spondylitis
  A   is less common but more severe in females
  B   presents as a severe oligoarthritis
  C   is associated with both HLA DW3 and HLA B27
  D   is associated with amyloidosis
  E   involves the sternoclavicular joints

16   Skeletal muscle pain is a recognized presenting symptom of
  A   muscular dystrophy
  B   Parkinson's disease
  C   muscle phosphorylase deficiency
  D   trichinosis
  E   myasthenia gravis

17   Characteristic features of mixed connective tissue disease include
  A   anti-DNA antibody
  B   glomerulonephritis
  C   hypocomplementaemia
  D   polyarthritis
  E   cerebral involvement

12	A	**True**	contrast rheumatoid arthritis with MCP and PIP joint involvement
	B	**True**	very similar to rheumatoid arthritis but persistently seronegative. An asymmetric oligo-arthritis also occurs
	C	**True**	
	D	**True**	may occur in association with psoriasis without peripheral joint involvement
	E	**False**	

13	A	**False**	hypertrophic spinal osteo-arthritis
	B	**False**	HLA B5 associated in Japan and Turkey
	C	**True**	} may cause reactive arthritis, HLA B27
	D	**True**	} found in 70–90%
	E	**False**	

14	A	**False**	male predominance (20:1); difficult to diagnose in women
	B	**True**	typical cutaneous lesions anywhere especially soles and palms
	C	**True**	urethritis is both a manifestation and a precipitating factor
	D	**True**	
	E	**True**	only 20% have no joint symptoms 1–5 years after onset

15	A	**False**	relatively equal sex ratio; more severe disease in young men
	B	**True**	affects spinal, sacro-iliac, hip and knee joints
	C	**False**	HLA B27. DW3 associated with rheumatoid arthritis
	D	**True**	a cause of renal failure
	E	**True**	

16	A	**False**	weakness is the usual presenting feature
	B	**True**	patients often complain of pain and stiffness
	C	**True**	McArdle's syndrome
	D	**True**	the female worm *Trichinella spiralis* discharges larvae which lodge in skeletal muscles
	E	**False**	muscle fatigue and weakness are typical

17	A	**False**	antibodies to extractable nuclear antigen and RNA
	B	**False**	involvement of the kidneys or brain is rare unlike SLE
	C	**False**	typical of SLE
	D	**True**	
	E	**False**	

18   Raynaud's phenomenon is an expected feature of
  A   rheumatoid arthritis
  B   shoulder–hand syndrome
  C   systemic lupus erythematosus
  D   polyarteritis nodosa
  E   mixed connective tissue disease

19   Neurological involvement in systemic lupus erythematosus
  A   affects peripheral nerves more commonly than the brain
  B   occurs as a presenting manifestation of SLE
  C   is usefully monitored by sequential EEG examination
  D   with diffuse CNS involvement confers a poor prognosis
  E   can manifest as a personality change

20   Skin changes in scleroderma characteristically include
  A   oedema
  B   telangiectasia
  C   hyperhydrosis
  D   hyperpigmentation
  E   localized plaques

21   Recognized features of dermatomyositis include
  A   purple discoloration over the dorsum of the fingers
  B   proximal myopathy
  C   a psoriasiform rash
  D   cutaneous vasculitis
  E   periorbital oedema

22   Immunological phenomena occurring in systemic lupus erythematosus include
  A   rheumatoid factor
  B   anti-DNA antibodies
  C   anti-mitochondrial antibody
  D   elevated serum complement C3 and C4
  E   IgG antibody to DNA histone

23   Characteristic features of polyarteritis nodosa include
  A   hepatobiliary infarction
  B   hypertension
  C   acute pancreatitis
  D   myocardial infarction
  E   neutrophil leucocytosis

18 A **True**   may precede arthritis by many years
    B **False**   vasomotor changes in wrist resemble Sudeck's
                   atrophy
    C **True**   less commonly seen in SLE than MCTD or
                   scleroderma
    D **False**   skin ulcers, digital vasculitis and gangrene are typical
                   but Raynaud's is unusual
    E **True**

19 A **False** ⎤ cerebral involvement, often mild in nature,
    B **True** ⎬ is common. The EEG is often abnormal even in the
    C **False** ⎦ absence of overt disease
    D **True**   except for seizures alone
    E **True**

20 A **True**   an early feature
    B **True**   characteristic
    C **False**
    D **True**
    E **True**   morphoea

21 A **True** ⎤
    B **True** ⎥
    C **True** ⎬ all characteristic features
    D **True** ⎥
    E **True** ⎦

22 A **True**   30–40%
    B **True**   both double and single stranded DNA antibodies
    C **True**   other cytoplasmic antibodies also
    D **False**   hypocomplementaemia
    E **True**   LE cell phenomenon

23 A **True**   necrotizing arteritis may produce infarcts in many
                   organs, especially kidneys, liver and bowel
    B **True**
    C **True**
    D **True**
    E **True**   leucocytosis reflects the severity of the disease

24 Osteoporosis
  A affects men more than women
  B associated fracture rates are reduced by vitamin D therapy
  C is a common feature of rheumatoid disease
  D bone histology shows an abnormal osteoid composition
  E is usually asymptomatic

25 Primary generalized osteo-arthrosis
  A involvement of the hands produces severe disability
  B causes ankylosis of the involved joints
  C affects men and women equally
  D characteristically involves the wrist joint
  E is often familial

26 Chondrocalcinosis is a recognized feature of
  A osteochondritis dissecans
  B haemochromatosis
  C hyperparathyroidism
  D pseudogout
  E gout

27 A 16-year-old boy presents with a 2-week history of a fever and a painful swollen ankle. The following statements are true
  A a normal X-ray excludes osteomyelitis
  B joint aspiration should be performed urgently
  C rheumatic fever is the likeliest cause if there is a tachycardia, systolic murmur and a third heart sound
  D a history of dysentery 1 month previously is likely to be significant
  E X-rays of the sacro-iliac joints should be performed

28 In gout
  A acute attacks are precipitated by weight reduction
  B thiazide diuretics will reduce the serum urate
  C olecranon bursitis is a recognized feature
  D pre-menopausal women are rarely affected
  E only joint aspiration with synovial fluid microscopy can prove the diagnosis

29 Allopurinol therapy
  A in combination with probenecid should be avoided
  B increases the serum cholesterol
  C is useful in gout resulting from renal failure
  D should be decreased in dosage when given with azathioprine therapy
  E precipitates acute gout

24   A   **False**
    B   **False**   only oestrogen therapy in women is useful
    C   **True**
    D   **False**   osteomalacia. All bone elements are reduced in osteoporosis
    E   **True**

---

25   A   **False**   although 60% of patients have hand involvement, disability is not severe
    B   **False**   fibrous ankylosis occurs in seronegative spondylo-arthritis, bony ankylosis in rheumatoid disease
    C   **False**   females are twice as likely to be affected especially post-menopausal women
    D   **False**   contrasts with rheumatoid disease
    E   **True**   40% have a family history

---

26   A   **False**   sclerosis of loose bodies and the joint margins
    B   **True**
    C   **True**
    D   **True**   usually seen in wrists, knees and symphysis pubis
    E   **False**

---

27   A   **False**   X-ray changes usually only occur after several weeks
    B   **True**   the best way of confirming infection and identifying the organism
    C   **False**   insufficient evidence (Duckett Jones criteria)
    D   **True**   usual time delay: 3–6 weeks
    E   **False**   sacro-iliac radiographs are seldom abnormal in this age group

---

28   A   **True**   usually only with severe calorie restriction
    B   **False**   thiazides increase serum urate and precipitate gout
    C   **True**   may be the only clinical feature
    D   **True**   also rare in eunuchs
    E   **True**   hyperuricaemia is characteristic but not pathognomonic nor always present

---

29   A   **False**   both act independently
    B   **False**
    C   **True**   reduces urate production
    D   **False**   purine metabolism is decreased, necessitating a lower dosage of azathioprine
    E   **True**   may provoke acute attacks due to inhibition of mono-oxygenase activity

30   Arthropathy is a recognized feature of
A   parvovirus B19 infection
B   *Yersinia* infection
C   type II hyperlipoproteinaemia
D   amyloidosis
E   prostatic carcinoma

31   A female with a 20-year history of erosive sero-positive rheumatoid arthritis is found to have a total WBC of $1.8 \times 10^9/l$, haemoglobin 10.5 g/dl and a mild thrombocytopenia. The following statements are correct
A   leg ulceration is a likely complication
B   the presence of a positive ANF suggests SLE rather than Felty's syndrome
C   splenectomy will improve the leucopenia
D   long-term prophylactic antibiotics are indicated
E   penicillamine therapy should be instituted

32   A male of 50 years presents with chronic back pain. Spinal X-rays show a decreased bone density with serum calcium 3.2 mmol/l and serum phosphate 0.82 mmol/l. The differential diagnoses include
A   renal osteodystrophy
B   myelomatosis
C   primary hyperparathyroidism
D   sarcoidosis
E   Paget's disease

33   Gouty tophi are found in the
A   pinna of the ears
B   fingertips, palms and soles of the feet
C   aortic and mitral valves
D   vocal cords, arytenoids and tongue
E   liver, spleen, lungs and brain

34   Causes of hyperuricaemia include
A   azapropazone
B   pyrazinamide
C   Waldenstrom's macroglobulinaemia
D   hypoxanthine-guanine phosphoribosyl transferase (HGPRT) deficiency
E   acute intermittent porphyria

30 A **True**   often a helpful diagnostic feature
    B **True**   reactive arthritis 3 weeks after infection usually affecting the lower limb joints
    C **True**   migratory relapsing and remitting arthritis
    D **True**   often resembling rheumatoid arthritis
    E **True**   may occur well before other manifestations of malignancy, the knees, ankles, MCP and MTP joints commonly affected

31 A **True**   Felty's syndrome is often associated with vasculitic leg ulcers
    B **False** ANF is common in Felty's syndrome
    C **False** no association between size of spleen and the haematological findings
    D **False** recurrent infections are unlikely with WBC > 0.8 × 10^9/l
    E **False** thrombocytopenia precludes such therapy

32 A **False** hyperphosphataemia and hypocalcaemia
    B **True**   hypercalcaemia confers a poor prognosis
    C **True**
    D **True**   increased sensitivity to vitamin D
    E **False** calcium and phosphate are normal

    Ca 2·12–2·65.
    Po₄ 2–0·8 – 1·45.

33 A **True**
    B **True**
    C **True** ⎱ tophi are found in the eye, tongue
    D **True** ⎰ larynx and heart on rare occasions
    E **False**

34 A **False** many NSAIDs have uricosuric properties
    B **True**   antituberculosis antibiotic that precipitates gout
    C **True**   increased turnover of purines
    D **True**   Lesch–Nyhan syndrome
    E **False** hypouricaemia

35   Useful second-line agents in the treatment of rheumatoid arthritis include
   A   sulphinpyrazone
   B   hydroxychloroquine
   C   azathioprine
   D   acetylsalicylic acid
   E   sodium aurothiomalate

36   In Wegener's granulomatosis
   A   serum anti-neutrophil cytoplasmic antibodies are typically present
   B   eosinophilia is a characteristic feature
   C   cyclophosphamide is a useful treatment
   D   oropharyngeal ulceration is characteristically destructive
   E   cavitating pulmonary lesions are recognized findings

37   In supraspinatus tendinitis
   A   nocturnal shoulder pain is characteristic
   B   resisted external rotation of shoulder typically increases pain
   C   calcification on X-ray is an indication for injected corticosteroid
   D   fever occurs in acute bursitis
   E   early active physiotherapy is the treatment of choice

38   Dupuytren's contracture
   A   results from chronic de Quervain's tenosynovitis
   B   is commoner in diabetes mellitus
   C   is a cause of carpal tunnel syndrome
   D   usually affects the 4th and 5th fingers
   E   affects the plantar fascia

39   Radiological features of rheumatoid arthritis include
   A   increased joint space
   B   reabsorption of terminal phalanges
   C   periarticular osteoporosis
   D   atlanto-axial subluxation
   E   aseptic necrosis of femoral head

40   Abnormalities of the hand on clinical examination in rheumatoid arthritis include
   A   trigger fingers
   B   extensor tendon rupture
   C   dorsal subluxation of ulna
   D   ulnar deviation of the metacarpophalangeal joints
   E   swellings over the dorsum of the distal interphalangeal joints

35 A **False** sulphasalazine
    B **True**   both chloroquine and hydroxychloroquine
    C **True**   useful if gold or penicillamine is ineffective
    D **False** like other NSAIDs, useful first-line treatment only
    E **True**   gold salt

36 A **True**   a significant ANCA titre is of diagnostic importance
    B **False** Churg–Strauss vasculitis
    C **True**
    D **True**   midline necrotizing granulomata occur
    E **True**

37 A **True**   with inability to lie on shoulder
    B **False** resisted abduction of shoulder
    C **False** calcification can be asymptomatic
    D **True**   pain, swelling and muscle spasm may mimic gout or
                   septic arthritis
    E **False** rest with local steroid/anaesthetic injection and oral
                   NSAIDs if necessary

38 A **False**
    B **True**   especially men
    C **False** the transverse carpal ligament compresses median
                   nerve
    D **True**   4th greater than 5th; 3rd, 2nd and 1st less commonly
    E **True**

39 A **False** joint space is lost due to synovial swelling
    B **False** more typical of psoriatic arthropathy
    C **True**
    D **True**
    E **True**   especially if oral corticosteroids have been used

40 A **True**   tenosynovitis of flexor tendons
    B **True**
    C **True**   inferior radio-ulnar arthritis
    D **True**
    E **False** Heberden's nodes seen in osteo-arthrosis

Psychiatry

1 **An organic basis for psychiatric symptoms is suggested by**
   A   disorientation in time and place
   B   auditory hallucinations
   C   visual hallucinations
   D   perseveration
   E   inability to recall distant events in time

2 **Obsessional behaviour is characteristically**
   A   repetitive
   B   attention seeking
   C   regarded as abnormal by the patient
   D   resisted by the patient
   E   unaccompanied by depression

3 **Early symptoms suggestive of schizophrenia include**
   A   early-morning waking
   B   loss of emotional responses
   C   visual hallucinations
   D   a feeling of being subjected to evil influences
   E   failure to recall recent events

4 **Amnesia is a recognized feature of**
   A   aspirin poisoning
   B   hysterical disorder
   C   schizophrenia
   D   head injury
   E   psychoneurotic disorders

5 **Korsakoff's psychosis is characterized by**
   A   impairment of long-term memory
   B   epileptic seizures
   C   peripheral neuropathy
   D   confabulation
   E   visual hallucinations

6 **Recognized features of alcohol dependence include**
   A   depression
   B   relief of withdrawal symptoms by alcohol ingestion
   C   relapses even after prolonged abstinence
   D   feelings of guilt about alcohol use
   E   decreased tolerance to alcohol

1 A **True**
   B **False**   more often occurs in schizophrenia and other
                   functional disorders
   C **True**   rarely in schizophrenia
   D **True**
   E **False**   short-term memory rather than long-term memory

2 A **True**   usually repetitive and regarded as abnormal by the
                   patient. Many patients are reluctant to talk about the
                   problem
   B **False**
   C **True**
   D **True**
   E **False**   it can progress to depression

3 A **False**   depression
   B **True**
   C **False**   hallucinations are usually auditory; visual
                   hallucinations are uncommon
   D **True**   passivity phenomena are common
   E **False**   dementia and organic brain syndromes

4 A **False**
   B **True**   characteristic of hysterical fugues
   C **False**
   D **True**   any organic brain disease including Alzheimer's
                   disease, Korsakoff's psychosis, post-traumatic,
                   vascular disease, encephalitis, carbon monoxide
                   poisoning, cerebral tumour and in epilepsy
                   especially of temporal lobe type
   E **False**

5 A **False**   short-term memory impaired
   B **False**   fits are usually a feature of alcohol withdrawal
   C **True**   'psychosis polyneuritica' in Korsakoff's original
                   description
   D **True**
   E **False**   feature of delirium tremens

6 A **True**   increased suicide risk especially in males
   B **True**
   C **True**
   D **True**
   E **True**   tolerance is increased initially then rapidly decreases
                   as the illness progresses

7 **Drugs associated with physical dependence include**
   A temazepam
   B amitriptyline
   C dihydrocodeine
   D cannabis resin
   E dexamphetamine sulphate

8 **Features of hysterical conversion disorder include**
   A apparent lack of concern
   B fugue states
   C pseudoseizures
   D manipulative behaviour
   E repeated hand-washing

9 **Factors associated with an increased risk of suicide after a suicide attempt include**
   A recent bereavement
   B alcohol abuse
   C preplanning
   D living alone away from home
   E female gender

10 **Under the Mental Health Act, 1983 (England and Wales), emergency detention of a patient already in hospital for a further 72 hours requires the signature of**
   A a state-registered nurse
   B the doctor in charge
   C a patient's relative
   D a police officer
   E a social worker

11 **Recognized features of Alzheimer's disease include**
   A a family history of dementia
   B sleep disturbance
   C extensor plantar responses
   D topographagnosia
   E dysarthria and dysphasia

12 **Somatic symptoms typical of depressive illness include**
   A dysmenorrhoea
   B constipation
   C anorexia
   D loss of libido
   E sweating

7 A **True**   use should be limited to short-term only
   B **False** may be required long-term to prevent relapse
   C **True**   all opiates are potentially addictive
   D **False**
· E **True**

---

8 A **True**   'belle indifference'
   B **False** hysterical dissociation
   C **True**
   D **False**
   E **False** obsessive compulsive disorder

---

9 A **True**   bereavement, unemployment, isolation and mental
                  illness
   B **True**   and drug addiction
   C **True**   for example, purchase of a gun or poison
   D **True**
   E **False** males are more at risk

---

10 A **False** ⎫
   B **True**   ⎪
   C **False** ⎬ section 5 (2) of the act requires only
   D **False** ⎪ the signature of the doctor in charge
   E **False** ⎭

---

11 A **True**   family history sometimes suggests an autosomal
                  dominant trait
   B **True**
   C **False** organic brain syndromes must be excluded
   D **True**   inability to find one's way in familiar surroundings
   E **True**

---

12 A **False** amenorrhoea is more likely
   B **True**
   C **True**
   D **True**
   E **False** more typical of anxiety

13 Features suggesting neurosis rather than psychosis include
    A grandiose delusions
    B lack of insight and awareness of a problem
    C depersonalization
    D cognitive impairment
    E monosymptomatic phobias with a family history of phobic disorder

14 Defence mechanisms against anxiety include
    A anger
    B denial
    C regression
    D idealization
    E dissociation

15 Abnormal illness behaviour is suggested by
    A a relentless search for an underlying disease
    B increased sense of responsibility for illness and its treatment
    C adoption of the sick role
    D disability disproportionate to signs and symptoms
    E obsession with health-promoting activities

16 Typical features of somatization disorders include
    A multiple, unexplained physical complaints
    B preoccupation with the fear of illness
    C onset of symptoms after the age of 30
    D previous history of unsuccessful surgical operations
    E conscious simulation of illness to obtain exemption from work

17 Useful drugs in the treatment of depression include
    A fluvoxamine
    B phenelzine
    C flurazepam
    D trifluperidol
    E sulpiride

18 Characteristic features of hypomania include
    A flight of ideas
    B rhyming speech
    C hypersomnia
    D weight gain
    E sexual promiscuity

19 Side-effects of lithium therapy include
    A improvement in psoriasis
    B fine tremor
    C nephrogenic diabetes insipidus
    D goitre
    E thyrotoxicosis

13 A **False** mania and GPI
    B **False** psychosis
    C **True**
    D **False**
    E **True** morbidity risk of 30% in first-degree relatives of patients with panic disorder

14 A **True** more often a defence against bereavement
    B **True** pretending fear does not exist
    C **True** becoming more childlike and demanding
    D **True**
    E **True**

15 A **True**
    B **False** abrogation of all responsibility for illness to the doctors
    C **True**
    D **True**
    E **False** avoidance of health-promoting roles and activities

16 A **True** often arising from early childhood
    B **True** hypochondriasis
    C **False** uncommon if not rare
    D **True** characteristic; especially appendicectomy and hysterectomy
    E **False** malingering

17 A **True** selective serotonin (5HT) re-uptake inhibitor
    B **True** reversibly inhibits monoamine oxidase
    C **False** long-acting hypnotic
    D **False** major tranquillizer
    E **False** used in schizophrenia

18 A **True**
    B **True**
    C **False** patients are typically restless, quick-witted, self-confident and usually need very little sleep
    D **False** may lose weight because they are too distracted to eat
    E **True**

19 A **False** psoriasis may be exacerbated
    B **True**
    C **True**
    D **True**
    E **False** inhibits thyroidal release of T4; hypothyroidism but induces symptoms akin to hyperthyroidism, namely nausea, anorexia, tremor and diarrhoea

20 Diagnostic features favouring anorexia nervosa rather than bulimia nervosa include

   A   weight loss and amenorrhoea
   B   obsessive fear of weight gain
   C   onset after the age of 25
   D   social withdrawal
   E   vomiting and purgation

20 A **True**   weight and menstruation are usually maintained in
                   bulimia
    B **False** typical of both disorders
    C **False** symptoms usually start as a teenager
    D **True**   bulimic patients are less introverted
    E **False** occur in both disorders

Dermatology/genito-urinary medicine/geriatrics/ophthalmology

1 **Scalp involvement is typical of the following dermatological disorders**
   A discoid lupus erythematosus
   B scabies
   C tylosis
   D psoriasis
   E erythrasma

2 **In exfoliative dermatitis**
   A there is often significant body protein loss
   B vesicles are rarely seen
   C atopic eczema is a predisposing condition
   D systemic corticosteroids are contraindicated
   E previous psoriasis is an aetiological factor

3 **Skin manifestations of visceral malignancy include**
   A erythema multiforme
   B pityriasis versicolor
   C dermatomyositis
   D acanthosis nigricans
   E acquired hypertrichosis lanuginosa

4 **In dermatitis herpetiformis**
   A uninvolved skin exhibits IgA deposits at the dermo-epidermal junction
   B there is 90% chance of spontaneous remission
   C dapsone treatment causes haemolytic anaemia in some patients
   D the mucous membranes are usually spared
   E partial or total villous atrophy occurs in 10–20% of patients

5 **Causes of blistering skin lesions include**
   A insect bites
   B porphyria cutanea tarda
   C allergic contact dermatitis
   D rosacea
   E pityriasis versicolor

1 A **True**   causes scarring alopecia
   B **False** finger webs, wrists and genitalia. Scalp and face
                 spared
   C **False** confined to palms and soles
   D **True**   causes adherent scaling
   E **False** *Corynebacterium minutissimum* infection affects toe
                 clefts, axillae and groins

2 A **True**   serum albumin falls due to skin loss and reduced
                 protein synthesis
   B **True**   redness, itch, oedema, scaling and heat predominate
   C **True**
   D **False** may be life-saving
   E **True**

3 A **False** infection, drugs, collagen, vascular diseases are the
                 causes
   B **False** commensal yeast infection
   C **True**   not as often as was previously thought
   D **True**   gastric adenocarcinoma or lymphoma especially
   E **True**   blonde downy hair over face associated with
                 Hodgkin's disease particularly

4 A **True**   usually IgA predominates
   B **False** chronic disorder
   C **True**
   D **False**
   E **False** occurs in 80–90%

5 A **True**   especially on lower legs
   B **True**   often on exposed areas of skin
   C **True**   healing to leave scars
   D **False**
   E **False**

6　Cutaneous ulceration is a recognized feature of
　A　polyarteritis nodosa
　B　dermatitis artefacta
　C　rheumatoid arthritis
　D　sickle-cell anaemia
　E　lupus pernio

7　A 60-year-old woman presents with a 3-month history of an itchy red rash involving the trunk and limbs. One week previously she had developed tense blisters on the lower limbs and trunk. Examination of the oral mucosa is normal. The following statements are correct
　A　the most likely diagnosis is bullous impetigo
　B　the absence of oral lesions favours pemphigus vulgaris
　C　biopsy of a lesion showing the presence of a subepidermal blister is compatible with bullous pemphigoid
　D　subepidermal blister formation also occurs in erythema multiforme
　E　a search should be made for underlying malignancy

8　The following statements about malignant melanoma are correct
　A　epidermal dendritic cell proliferation is uncontrolled
　B　nodular melanoma has a better prognosis than malignant lentigo
　C　onset before puberty is rare
　D　most arise from a pre-existing pigmented naevus
　E　the presence of pigment distinguishes melanomas from basal cell carcinomas

9　Recognized causes of a lichenoid eruption include
　A　penicillin
　B　aspirin
　C　graft-versus-host disease
　D　gold
　E　quinine

10　Useful treatments for psoriasis include
　A　isotretinoin
　B　cyclosporin
　C　methotrexate
　D　psoralen combined with UVA therapy
　E　dapsone

11　Diseases with a sexual mode of transmission include
　A　molluscum contagiosum
　B　scabies
　C　trichinosis
　D　herpes zoster
　E　anisakiasis

6 A **True**   due to cutaneous vasculitis
   B **True**   self-inflicted skin lesion with irregular, bizarre
               configurations
   C **True**   especially Felty's syndrome
   D **True**   usually on lower limbs
   E **False** dusky infiltrated plaques on nose and fingers in
               sarcoidosis

7 A **False**
   B **False** 60% of patients with pemphigus vulgaris present
               with oral lesions
   C **True**
   D **True**   the bullous form of erythema multiforme
   E **False**

8 A **True**   melanocytes are dendritic cells in basal layers of
               epidermis
   B **False** prognosis worse with increasing depth of lesion
   C **True**
   D **False** around 50% arise spontaneously
   E **False** basal cell carcinoma can be pigmented

9 A **False** morbilliform eruptions
   B **False** urticarial rashes
   C **True**   lichen planus eruptions are papular, often itchy and
               may involve the mucous membranes and the nails
   D **True**
   E **True**

10 A **False** used in acne vulgaris
   B **True**
   C **True**
   D **True**   PUVA (photochemotherapy)
   E **False** dermatitis herpetiformis

11 A **True**
   B **True**
   C **False** nematode in pork products
   D **False** herpes simplex
   E **False** nematode in raw fish

12   Skin lesions in secondary syphilis include
  A   patchy alopecia
  B   condylomata acuminata
  C   hypopigmented anaesthetic lesion
  D   erythroderma
  E   scaling rash on soles

13   In gonorrhoea, the following statements are correct
  A   the majority of affected females are asymptomatic
  B   bloody rectal discharge is a recognized presentation
  C   infection in pregnancy has low perinatal mortality
  D   Gram-negative extracellular diplococci are seen on
      microscopy
  E   acute septic arthritis is a recognized complication

14   In non-specific urethritis (NSU)
  A   amoxycillin is the treatment of choice
  B   *Chlamydia trachomatis* accounts for the majority of cases
  C   prostatitis is a late complication
  D   urethral smears show a lymphocytic predominance
  E   haematosperma is a characteristic feature

15   Features of a primary syphilitic chancre include
  A   appearance as a bleeding anal fissure
  B   associated lymphadenitis
  C   spontaneous healing within 4 weeks
  D   erosive, painful lesion on a finger
  E   a painless ulcerated papule on the lip

16   Complications of genital herpes simplex (HSV-2) infection include
  A   diarrhoea
  B   encephalitis
  C   neonatal intrapartum infection
  D   urinary retention
  E   congenital transplacental infection

17   Painless progressive visual loss is a feature of
  A   central retinal artery occlusion
  B   retinitis pigmentosa
  C   senile macular degeneration
  D   cranial arteritis
  E   retinoblastoma

18   Orbital oedema is a typical feature of
  A   IIIrd cranial nerve palsy
  B   cavernous sinus thrombosis
  C   South American trypanosomiasis
  D   hypoparathyroidism
  E   dermatomyositis

12 A **True**
    B **False** genital warts, condylomata lata are typical
    C **False** a feature of tuberculoid leprosy
    D **False** generalized exfoliative dermatitis
    E **True** resembles psoriasis

13 A **True** around 70%
    B **True** usually homosexuals
    C **False** may cause abortion or premature labour
    D **True** both intra- and extracellular Gram-negative
             diplococci seen
    E **True** commoner in females

14 A **False** tetracycline or erythromycin
    B **True** 50% of patients with NSU
    C **True**
    D **False** polymorph leucocytes
    E **False**

15 A **True** many chancres do not arise on the genitalia and not
             all are painless or ulcerated
    B **True**
    C **True**
    D **True** dark-ground microscopy of serum from chancre
             reveals *Treponema pallidum*
    E **True**

16 A **True** herpetic proctitis
    B **True** often after neonatal infection
    C **True**
    D **True** sacral radiculopathy
    E **True** rare; may produce microcephaly and chorioretinitis

17 A **False** sudden loss of vision
    B **True**
    C **True**
    D **False** sudden irreversible blindness
    E **True** visual loss (bilateral in 30%); 90% present under the
             age of 3

18 A **False** ptosis but not oedema
    B **True**
    C **True**
    D **False** although cataract occurs
    E **True** lilac discoloration of eyelids

19   Characteristic features of chronic simple (open-angle) glaucoma include
  A   painful red eye
  B   optic atrophy
  C   diminished peripheral vision
  D   cupping of optic disc
  E   normal visual acuity

20   Chorioretinitis is a recognized complication of
  A   measles
  B   gonorrhoea
  C   toxoplasmosis
  D   cytomegalovirus infection
  E   tuberculosis

21   Anterior uveitis is a typical feature of
  A   systemic lupus erythematosus
  B   sarcoidosis
  C   herpes zoster infection
  D   Whipple's disease
  E   toxocariasis

22   Associations of retinal soft exudates include
  A   HIV infection
  B   high lipid content of the lesion
  C   pre-proliferative diabetic retinopathy
  D   Marfan's syndrome
  E   vitamin A deficiency

23   Granuloma inguinale (donovanosis) is
  A   due to a chlamydial infection
  B   a cause of multiple genital lesions
  C   best diagnosed by the Frei skin test
  D   a cause of false-positive serological tests for syphilis
  E   effectively treated with penicillin

24   Features favouring the diagnosis of multi-infarct dementia rather than Alzheimer's disease include
  A   memory loss as a prominent early feature
  B   abnormal EEG
  C   stepwise deterioration in mental function
  D   personality change before any significant intellectual deterioration
  E   Parkinsonian features

19 A **False**   acute closed-angle glaucoma
    B **True**
    C **True**
    D **True**
    E **False**   there is usually some visual loss; treatment should prevent progression

20 A **False**
    B **False**
    C **True**   } intrauterine infections, also syphilis
    D **True**   }
    E **True**   choroidal tubercles in miliary TB heal producing choroiditis

21 A **False**   scleritis and episcleritis
    B **True**
    C **True**
    D **False**   papillitis or choroiditis
    E **False**   low-grade <u>posterior</u> uveitis

22 A **True**   cotton wool spots seen at any stage of HIV infection
    B **False**   <u>hard</u> exudates
    C **True**   indicators of severe retinal ischaemia
    D **False**   dislocated lens is usual eye feature
    E **False**   keratomalacia

23 A **False**   *Calymmatobacterium granulomatis* (a Gram-negative *Klebsiella*-like organism)
    B **True**
    C **False**   a skin test for hypersensitivity to *Chlamydia*
    D **False**
    E **False**   tetracycline, co-trimoxazole, streptomycin

24 A **False**   more likely in Alzheimer's disease
    B **False**   abnormal EEGs can occur in both
    C **True**
    D **True**   frontal lobe infarct(s)
    E **False**   Parkinsonian features are common in both disorders

25   Recognized features of hypothermia in the elderly include
A   muscle rigidity
B   hypoglycaemia
C   elevated serum aspartate aminotransferase
D   tachypnoea
E   atrial fibrillation

26   Normal clinical findings in healthy elderly subjects include
A   a third heart sound
B   impaired proprioception
C   basal lung crepitations
D   upbeat nystagmus
E   absent ankle jerks

27   Postural hypotension is a recognized feature of
A   chlorpromazine therapy
B   diabetic autonomic neuropathy
C   Shy–Drager syndrome
D   rising from bed after prolonged illness
E   vitamin E deficiency

28   Biochemical changes in the blood associated with normal ageing include
A   elevated alkaline phosphatase
B   elevated creatinine kinase
C   low serum ferritin
D   low serum albumin
E   low serum FSH in females

29   Urinary incontinence is potentially reversible in the following disorders
A   faecal impaction
B   normal pressure hydrocephalus
C   immobility secondary to Parkinson's disease
D   detrusor instability
E   multiple sclerosis

30   Acute confusional states in the elderly are a recognized feature of
A   laxative therapy
B   anticholinergic drug therapy
C   pneumonia
D   hypoglycaemia
E   subdural haematoma

25 A **True** can cause neck stiffness
   B **True** both hypo- and hyperglycaemia are recognized
   C **True** and hyperamylasaemia
   D **False** respirations are slow and shallow
   E **True** abnormalities of cardiac rhythm are common

26 A **False** indicates heart disease
   B **False** impaired vibration is common
   C **False** underlying cardiac or respiratory disease
   D **False** indicates brain stem disease
   E **True** if bilateral and symmetrical

27 A **True** an alpha-adrenergic receptor blocker
   B **True**
   C **True** progressive autonomic failure
   D **True**
   E **False**

28 A **False**
   B **False**
   C **False** } all indicate underlying disorders irrespective of age
   D **False**
   E **False**

29 A **True**
   B **True**
   C **True**
   D **True**
   E **False**

30 A **False**
   B **True** many drugs with effects within the CNS
   C **True** any severe infection
   D **True** especially long-acting sulphonylureas
   E **True** this is more likely to cause chronic confusion

Basic sciences (including statistics)

1   **Autosomal dominant inheritance is a characteristic feature of**
    A   Gilbert's syndrome
    B   limb girdle muscular dystrophy
    C   cystic fibrosis
    D   achondroplasia
    E   Charcot–Marie–Tooth disease

2   **Autosomal recessive inheritance is a characteristic feature of**
    A   hereditary haemorrhagic telangiectasia
    B   hereditary spherocytosis
    C   Wilson's disease
    D   phenylketonuria
    E   pseudohypoparathyroidism

3   **In X-linked recessive inheritance**
    A   half of the sons of a carrier female are carriers
    B   all daughters of affected males are carriers
    C   all sons of an affected male are normal
    D   there is a 1-in-4 chance of a child of a female carrier being affected
    E   heterozygous females are unaffected

4   **Useful methods of preventing genetic disease include**
    A   avoidance of consanguinity
    B   pre-implantation diagnosis and genetic counselling
    C   sterilization
    D   maternal alpha-fetoprotein measurement
    E   transabdominal chorionic villus biopsy

5   **Methods of gene delivery in gene therapy include**
    A   retrovirus carriage
    B   tissue bombardment with biolistic devices
    C   direct DNA uptake
    D   liposomal carriage
    E   adenovirus carriage

1 A **True**
  B **False** autosomal recessive affecting pelvis and/or shoulder girdle muscles particularly
  C **False** autosomal recessive
  D **True** predominantly new mutations
  E **True** this is hereditary motor and sensory neuropathy (HMSN) type II

2 A **False** autosomal dominant (Rendu–Osler–Weber syndrome)
  B **False** usually autosomal dominant affecting 1–2 per 10 000
  C **True** chromosome 13 defect causing hepato-lenticular degeneration
  D **True** deficiency of phenylalanine hydroxylase
  E **False** X-linked dominant mode of inheritance predominates

3 A **False** 50% of daughters are carriers. 50% of sons are affected
  B **True**
  C **True** because only the X chromosome is passed to daughters
  D **True** 1 in 2 chance of being boy with 50% chance of being affected
  E **True**

4 A **True**
  B **True** blastomere removal with DNA analysis
  C **True**
  D **True** screen at 16–19 weeks' gestation for neural tube defects (high level) or Down's syndrome (low level)
  E **True** with DNA probes, single gene defects can be identified

5 A **True** ⎫ high-energy bombardment with
  B **True** ⎪ biolistic devices can get DNA into
  C **True** ⎬ certain tissues, e.g. mammary gland.
  D **True** ⎪ Muscle can take up DNA directly and liposomes,
  E **True** ⎭ like viruses, are used for gene delivery

6   **Abnormalities leading to the breakage or rearrangement of chromosomes include**
   A   centromere banding
   B   reduction division
   C   deletion
   D   reciprocal translocation
   E   pericentric inversion

7   **Characteristic features of Klinefelter's syndrome include**
   A   psychopathic behaviour
   B   sterility
   C   normal sized testes
   D   gynaecomastia
   E   skin hyperpigmentation

8   **In man**
   A   somatic cell nuclei contain 22 pairs of homologous autosomes
   B   gamete nuclei are haploid with a single X or Y chromosome
   C   the X chromosome is smaller than the Y chromosome
   D   an F body in somatic cell nuclei represents a Y chromosome
   E   a Barr body is a genetically inactive X chromosome

9   **The arithmetic mean of a series of measurements is**
   A   the most commonly occurring value
   B   the value intermediate between the highest and lowest measurement
   C   twice the median
   D   the average value of all the measurements
   E   the sum of values of measurement multiplied by the number of measurements

10   **The following statements about a normal Gaussian distribution are correct**
   A   considerable skew of the values exists
   B   the mode and median coincide with the mean
   C   95% of the area under the curve is represented by the mean plus or minus one standard deviation
   D   the standard error of the mean is the standard deviation of the mean divided by the square root of the number of observations
   E   all people in the sample are normal

6 A **False** a staining technique for chromosomes
  B **False** meiosis in the production of gametes
  C **True** loss of material from either the long or short arm of a chromosome
  D **True** exchange of material between two non-identical chromosomes
  E **True** inversion of a segment of chromosome involving the centromere

---

7 A **False** karyotype 47 xyy
  B **True**
  C **False** testes are small
  D **True**
  E **False**

---

8 A **True** there are also two sex chromosomes
  B **True**
  C **False**
  D **True** fluorescent spots on interphase nuclei of male cells and represent Y chromosomes
  E **True**

---

9 A **False** this is the mode
  B **False**
  C **False**
  D **True**
  E **False**

---

10 A **False** non-skewed or parametric data
   B **True** the mode is the value that occurs most frequently; the median is the middle value of the range
   C **False** 95% is mean plus or minus <u>two</u> standard deviations
   D **True**
   E **False**

11   The Student's 't' test

   A   was developed specifically for use by students
   B   is a useful method of comparing two normally distributed samples
   C   requires reference tables for statistical assessment of the 't' value
   D   requires calculation of the standard error of the differences between two means
   E   uses the concepts of degrees of freedom and confidence limits

12   In the study of the relationship between weight and blood pressure in a sample group of individuals, useful statistical techniques would include

   A   analysis of variance
   B   correlation coefficient
   C   Student's 't' distribution
   D   the chi-square test
   E   regression analysis

13   In a double-blind, placebo-controlled, cross-over trial of a new drug for treating obesity

   A   the researcher does not know the treatment assigned to each patient volunteer
   B   an inadequate sample size can be the reason for not recognizing treatment superiority
   C   randomization safeguards against selection bias
   D   the trial should be stopped if one patient dies
   E   over 2000 patients are needed to show a therapeutic effect

14   In the chi-square test

   A   comparisons between groups are sought
   B   if small numbers are present, the test is more useful
   C   requires prior calculation of the potency ratio
   D $P < 0.001$ indicates statistical significance
   E   actual values, rather than the number of occurrences, are compared

15   Essential amino acids include

   A   leucine
   B   glycine
   C   tryptophan
   D   methionine
   E   glutamine

11 A **False** pseudonym of the mathematician, William Gosset
    B **True**
    C **True**
    D **True**
    E **True** 95% confidence limits = (1.96 × standard error) less than and greater than the mean

12 A **False** multiple comparison procedure when more than two variables are being assessed
    B **True** relationship between two variables
    C **False** comparison of two means and their standard deviations
    D **False** comparison of proportions (see below)
    E **True** prediction of the weight from a knowledge of the blood pressure

13 A **True** neither the patient nor researcher know
    B **True** type II error
    C **True**
    D **False** patient may be on placebo, although code for that patient should be broken
    E **False** depends on the degree of weight change in the group

14 A **True** the null hypothesis that there is no difference between groups is being tested
    B **False** often Yates correction required if numbers < 40 and this reduces value of chi-square
    C **False**
    D **True** any chance less than 1 in 20 ($P < 0.05$)
    E **False** the test is designed to compare proportions rather than actual values

15 A **True** ⎫
    B **False** ⎬ the eight essential amino acids are
    C **True** ⎬ methionine, lysine, tryptophan, phenylalanine
    D **True** ⎬ leucine, isoleucine, threonine and valine
    E **False** ⎭

16   Acetyl coenzyme A
A   inhibits conversion from pyruvate to oxaloacetic acid in the mitochondrion
B   inhibits its own production from pyruvate in the mitochondrion
C   inhibits glucose-6-phosphate production from fructose-6-phosphate in the cell cytoplasm
D   conversion to fatty acids is an energy-consuming action
E   production from citrate is enhanced in the fasting state

17   The constituents of very-low-density lipoprotein (VLDL) include
A   triacylglyceride
B   apolipoprotein A-II
C   cholesterol
D   phospholipid
E   chylomicrons

18   Gram-negative diplococci include
A   *Neisseria meningitidis*
B   *Streptococcus pneumoniae*
C   *Neisseria gonorrhoeae*
D   *Staphylococcus aureus*
E 〉 *Corynebacterium diphtheriae*

19   Arboviruses are responsible for the following infections
A   St Louis encephalitis
B   Omsk haemorrhagic fever
C   pharyngoconjunctival fever
D   Bornholm disease
E   hand, foot and mouth disease

20   An immunofluorescent technique is the basis of
A   testing for factor VIII antigen in haemophilia
B   the Rose–Waaler test
C   the TPHA test in syphilis
D   identification of tumour-specific antigens in sera
E   detection of tissue immunoglobulins

21   Immunoglobulins
A   are secreted by transformed T lymphocytes
B   produced by the lamina propria of the gut are IgA
C   crossing the placenta include IgM
D   on the surface of immature B lymphocytes include IgD
E   involved in immune complex formation include IgG

16 A **False** acetyl CoA is the starting point of Kreb's energy-producing cycle with production of oxaloacetate
    B **True**
    C **True** glucose-6-phosphate and fructose-6-phosphate are freely convertible but acetyl CoA promotes glucose-6-phosphate production to promote glycolysis
    D **True** as opposed to energy-producing
    E **False** acetyl CoA is formed from the oxidative decarboxylation of <u>pyruvate</u>

17 A **True** about 60% of VLDL
    B **False** this is constituent of HDL
    C **True** about 5% of VLDL
    D **True** about 14% of VLDL
    E **False** this is another type of lipoprotein

18 A **True**
    B **False** Gram-positive streptococci
    C **True**
    D **False** Gram-positive coccus
    E **False** Gram-positive bacillus

19 A **True** ⎫ arboviruses (arthropod borne) are usually
    B **True** ⎭ togaviruses borne by mosquitoes, ticks or flies
    C **False** adenovirus
    D **False** coxsackievirus B
    E **False** coxsackievirus A

20 A **False** ⎫
    B **False** ⎪ immunofluorescence is a technique for assessing
    C **False** ⎬ cell and tissue structures to identify and
    D **False** ⎪ localize particulate proteins such as
    E **True** ⎭ immunoglobulins

21 A **False** from transformed B lymphocytes, i.e. plasma cells
    B **True** IgA also produced in respiratory tract
    C **False** IgG is the only immunoglobulin which crosses the placenta
    D **True**
    E **True**

22   In the complement system

    A   only the classical pathway produces both C3 and C5 convertase

    B   components of the classical pathway are mainly beta-globulins

    C   the classical pathway is triggered by bacterial endotoxin

    D   the alternative pathway is triggered by platelet aggregation

    E   C1 esterase deficiency produces angio-oedema

23   Aetiological factors in the development of autoimmune disorders include

    A   loss of suppressor T cell control of T helper cell

    B   immunological exposure to sequestrated antigens

    C   bacterial mimicry of tissue antigen producing cross-reaction

    D   drug-induced immune complexes activating complement

    E   genetic variations in the major histocompatibility complex

24   Molecular abnormalities associated with acute myeloid leukaemia include

    A   N-ras mutation

    B   RBI gene

    C   tal-1 gene

    D   abnormal expression of c-*myc*

    E   altered expression of p53 gene

25   In molecular genetics, the following events occur in the cell nucleus rather than in the cytoplasm

    A   transcription to mRNA precursor

    B   cleaving of polypeptide chain

    C   translation of mRNA to gene product

    D   excision of introns and splicing of exons

    E   control of gene expression

26   Growth factors involved in normal haemopoiesis include

    A   erythropoietin

    B   granulocyte colony stimulation factor

    C   B interferon

    D   interleukin 1

    E   tumour necrosis factor

27   Cell receptors which activate adenylate cyclase include

    A   insulin

    B   alpha-2 adrenergic

    C   histamine 1

    D   thromboxane A2

    E   thyroid-stimulating hormone

22 A **False**   both classical and alternative pathways produce C3
                     convertase
    B **True**   synthesized in liver
    C **False** ⎱ alternative pathway. Classical pathway
    D **False** ⎰ triggered when immune complex combines with C1q
    E **True**

23 A **True**
    B **True**
    C **True**   streptococci and rheumatic fever
    D **True**   for example, antinuclear antibodies
    E **True**

24 A **True**   a proto-oncogene that controls the proliferation and
                     differentiation of many types of cell
    B **True**   an anti-oncogene suppressing tumour function. Both
                     N-ras mutation and the RBI gene are common in
                     AML
    C **False**   also known as SCL gene and is an oncogene fusion
                     gene seen in acute lymphoblastic leukaemia
    D **False**   this gene is sometimes dysregulated in ALL
    E **True**   an anti-oncogene that controls apoptosis and the
                     transcription of other genes

25 A **True**   direct copying of one strand of DNA occurs in all
                     nuclei
    B **False**   a cytoplasmic event
    C **False**   a cytoplasmic event
    D **True**   forms the processed mRNA
    E **True**

26 A **True**
    B **True**
    C **False**   antiviral cytokine
    D **True**
    E **False**

27 A **False**   intrinsic protein tyrosine kinase activity
    B **False**   inhibits adenylate cyclase
    C **False** ⎱ histamine 2 and prostacyclin
    D **False** ⎰ activate adenylate cyclase
    E **True**

28 **Proto-oncogene c-*myc* is associated with**
   A   colon carcinoma
   B   breast carcinoma
   C   cervical carcinoma
   D   small-cell lung carcinoma
   E   Burkitt's lymphoma

29 **Paraneoplastic syndromes are associated with the following ectopically produced hormones**
   A   cortisol
   B   prolactin
   C   osteoclast-activating factor (OAF)
   D   human chorionic gonadotrophin (HCG)
   E   erythropoietin

30 **Inherited conditions predisposing to malignant disease include**
   A   polyposis coli
   B   tuberous sclerosis
   C   beta-thalassaemia
   D   Turcot's syndrome
   E   tylosis palmaris et plantaris

31 **Recognized complications of radiotherapy include**
   A   squamous carcinoma of skin
   B   cataract
   C   leucopenia
   D   skin ulceration
   E   acute interstitial nephritis

32 **The incidence of a disease is**
   A   the number of cases of disease present at any given time in the sample under study
   B   a measure of both clinical and subclinical cases
   C   greater than the prevalence in chronic diseases
   D   a useful measure in determining the cause of a disease
   E   best determined from post-mortem data

33 **Recommendations of the UK National Advisory Committee on Nutrition Education (NACNE) include**
   A   reduction of dietary saturated fat to less than 35% of energy intake
   B   increase in dietary fibre to above 25 g/day
   C   increase polyunsaturated fat to greater than 5% of energy intake
   D   energy intake to achieve a body mass index (BMI) of between 25 and 30
   E   maintain a salt intake of 400 mmoles per day

28 A **False** c-*ras*
    B **True**
    C **True**
    D **True**
    E **True**

29 A **False** ACTH produced by small-cell lung carcinomas, producing hypokalaemic alkalosis but not Cushingoid appearance
    B **True**   renal carcinoma
    C **True**   myeloma causing hypercalcaemia
    D **True**   small-cell lung tumour causing gynaecomastia
    E **True**   cerebellar haemangioblastoma and uterine fibromyomata

30 A **True**   colonic carcinoma
    B **True**   glioma
    C **False**
    D **True**   colonic carcinoma and tumours of the brain and spinal cord
    E **True**   oesophageal carcinoma

31 A **True**
    B **True**
    C **True**
    D **True**
    E **True**

32 A **False** prevalence. Incidence is the number of new cases arising each year
    B **True**
    C **False**
    D **True**
    E **False**

33 A **False** total fat to less than 35%. Saturated fat to less than 15% of energy intake
    B **True**
    C **True**
    D **False** healthy BMI is between 20 and 25. Body mass index is weight (kg)/height (m)^2
    E **False** a reduction in salt intake is advised

34 **Metabolic changes associated with obesity include**
   A decreased glucose tolerance
   B increased insulin sensitivity
   C increased plasma triglycerides
   D increased fasting plasma insulin
   E decreased urinary 17-hydroxycorticoid excretion

35 **A decrease in oxygen affinity is seen in**
   A diabetic ketoacidosis
   B residence at high altitude
   C anaemia
   D blood transfusion
   E Eisenmenger's syndrome

36 **Free fatty acid release from adipose tissue is**
   A increased by noradrenaline
   B decreased by insulin
   C decreased by glucocorticoids
   D decreased by growth hormone
   E dependent on activated pancreatic lipase

37 **Acetylcholine is an excitatory parasympathetic neurotransmitter found in**
   A the smooth muscle of the bronchioles
   B the lacrimal glands
   C the detrusor muscle of the bladder
   D the erectile arterioles of the penis
   E the pyloric sphincter of the stomach

38 **Normal cerebro-spinal fluid**
   A is under a greater hydrostatic pressure than the venous sinuses of brain
   B is present within the subdural space
   C communicates from the lateral ventricle to the IIIrd ventricle via the foramen of Munro
   D has a volume of 500 ml in man
   E is produced in the arachnoid villi

39 **In the normal human liver**
   A the portal tracts lie at the periphery of hepatic lobules
   B the sinusoids flow into the central vein
   C 50% of hepatic oxygen requirements is supplied via the portal vein
   D Kupffer cells detoxify drugs in the circulation
   E hepatic lymph, formed in the space of Disse, accounts for half of the thoracic duct lymph flow

34 A True
   B False there is increased insulin resistance
   C True
   D True
   E False increased

---

35 A True ⎤
   B True ⎥ acidosis, hypoxia and anaemia shift the oxygen
   C True ⎦ dissociation curve to the right
   D False a marked fall in 2,3-DPG is seen with shift in O_2
            dissociation curve
   E True

---

36 A True rapidly as happens in fear or cold
   B True rapidly as blood glucose rises
   C False increased slowly, in response to stress
   D False increased slowly, in response to hunger
   E False dependent on activated <u>lipoprotein</u> lipase

---

37 A True
   B True secretomotor control
   C True bladder contraction
   D False vasodilation of arterioles due to <u>inhibitory</u> action
   E False relaxation of sphincteric muscle due to <u>inhibitory</u>
            action

---

38 A True
   B False subarachnoid space
   C True
   D False 120–150 ml
   E False produced in choroid plexuses. Arachnoid villi
            reabsorb

---

39 A True
   B True
   C True hepatic artery supplies one-third of total hepatic
            blood flow
   D False part of mononuclear phagocytic system. Hepatocytes
            detoxify
   E False

40 In the spinal cord

   A the dorsal columns predominantly convey pain and temperature sensation

   B spinothalamic fibres from the sacral segments lie innermost

   C the cauda equina begins at the level of the first sacral vertebra

   D the anterior spinal artery supplies the sensory compartments

   E the dorsal root ganglion lies within the subarachnoid space

40 A **False** vibration and proprioception
    B **False**
    C **False** spinal cord ends at the first lumbar vertebra
    D **False** supplies principally the anterior (motor) components
    E **False**

Mock MRCP Part 1

Answer ALL of the following 60 questions

Mark T, F or D against each of the 300 responses (T = true, F = false, D = don't know)

Remember, marks are deducted only for wrong answers. Time allowed: 2½ hours

1 **The ulnar nerve supplies**
   A the thenar muscles
   B all interossei
   C the first and second lumbricals
   D adductor pollicis
   E abductor pollicis brevis

2 **Elevation of the plasma gamma glutamyl transferase is a typical feature of**
   A osteomalacia
   B intrahepatic cholestasis
   C pregnancy
   D myocardial infarction
   E alcoholic hepatitis

3 **Elevated levels of serum immunoglobulin A (IgA) are usually seen in**
   A ankylosing spondylitis
   B polymyositis
   C dermatitis herpetiformis
   D chronic active hepatitis
   E primary biliary cirrhosis

4 **Autosomal recessive inheritance is characteristic of**
   A hereditary haemorrhagic telangiectasia
   B hereditary spherocytosis
   C Wilson's disease
   D phenylketonuria
   E pseudohypoparathyroidism

5 **The typical features of background diabetic retinopathy include**
   A venous irregularity
   B rubeosis iriditis
   C soft exudates
   D flame haemorrhages
   E disciform macular scar

1 A **True**
   B **True**
   C **False**
   D **True**
   E **False**

2 A **False**
   B **True**
   C **False**
   D **False**
   E **True**

3 A **True**
   B **False**
   C **False**
   D **True**
   E **False**

4 A **False**
   B **False**
   C **True**
   D **True**
   E **False**

5 A **True**
   B **False**
   C **False**
   D **False**
   E **False**

6   In a set of values
- **A**   the mode is that value which occurs most frequently
- **B**   the median is the mid-point on the scale of measurement above which lie exactly half the values
- **C**   having a normal distribution, the arithmetic mean, the mode and median coincide
- **D**   of a normally distributed variable, the probability of attaining a value higher than two standard deviations above the mean is approximately 1 in 40
- **E**   having a normal distribution, approximately 95% of values will be within the range between (mean plus 2 standard deviations) and (mean minus 2 standard deviations)

7   Complications of gonorrhoea in females include
- **A**   proctitis
- **B**   bartholinitis
- **C**   acute salpingitis
- **D**   optic atrophy
- **E**   perihepatitis

8   The use of the following drugs should be avoided in breast-feeding mothers
- **A**   propranolol
- **B**   aspirin
- **C**   metoclopramide
- **D**   salazopyrine
- **E**   thyroxine

9   Recognized features of acute lead poisoning include
- **A**   convulsions
- **B**   renal tubular dysfunction
- **C**   abdominal pain
- **D**   diarrhoea
- **E**   an erythematous rash

10   Failure of contraception in women taking a combined oral contraceptive steroid may result from coexistent use of
- **A**   vitamin C tablets
- **B**   carbamazepine
- **C**   rifampicin
- **D**   co-trimoxazole
- **E**   amitriptyline

11   Drugs which significantly inhibit hepatic mono-oxygenase activity include
- **A**   cimetidine
- **B**   phenytoin
- **C**   metronidazole
- **D**   spironolactone
- **E**   allopurinol

6 A **True**
   B **True**
   C **True**
   D **True**
   E **True**

7 A **True**
   B **True**
   C **True**
   D **False**
   E **True**

8 A **False**
   B **True**
   C **False**
   D **False**
   E **False**

9 A **True**
   B **True**
   C **True**
   D **False**
   E **False**

10 A **False**
    B **True**
    C **True**
    D **True**
    E **False**

11 A **True**
    B **False**
    C **True**
    D **False**
    E **True**

12   Characteristic features of severe paracetamol poisoning include
  A   hypoglycaemia
  B   renal failure
  C   metabolic acidosis
  D   hyperpyrexia
  E   hypotension

13   In renal failure due to myeloma
  A   glomerular damage is unusual
  B   intravenous urography is a useful investigation
  C   corticosteroid drugs are contraindicated
  D   haemodialysis is of no therapeutic value
  E   prognosis for patient survival is poor

14   Recognized problems after renal transplantation include
  A   hypercalcaemia
  B   lymphocele
  C   recurrent urinary tract infection
  D   metabolic alkalosis
  E   obstructive jaundice

15   In unilateral renal artery stenosis
  A   angiotensin-converting enzyme inhibitors are contraindicated
  B   arterial reconstructive surgery is the treatment of choice
  C   the affected kidney is usually larger than the unaffected one
  D   the contralateral kidney may develop amyloid
  E   an audible bruit is often absent

16   In membranous glomerulonephritis
  A   hypertension and renal failure are typically present at presentation
  B   cyclophosphamide treatment is often helpful
  C   diffuse deposits of C3 complement are seen in glomerular capillary walls
  D   patients usually present with macroscopic haematuria
  E   there is an increased incidence of thrombotic events

17   Hepatitis B virus infection
  A   rarely progresses to a chronic carrier state when acquired in the perinatal period
  B   is the commonest cause of post-transfusion hepatitis
  C   is not excluded by the absence of hepatitis-B surface antigen or antibody in serum
  D   should be treated with alpha interferon
  E   is decreasing in frequency in the Western world

12 A **True**
    B **True**
    C **True**
    D **False**
    E **True**

13 A **False**
    B **False**
    C **False**
    D **False**
    E **True**

14 A **True**
    B **True**
    C **True**
    D **False**
    E **False**

15 A **False**
    B **False**
    C **False**
    D **False**
    E **True**

16 A **True**
    B **False**
    C **True**
    D **False**
    E **True**

17 A **False**
    B **False**
    C **True**
    D **False**
    E **True**

18   In patients with the human immunodeficiency virus (HIV)
    A   diarrhoea due to cryptosporidiosis responds to metronidazole
    B   the development of oesophageal candidiasis is typical of the acquired immune deficiency syndrome (AIDS)
    C   Kaposi's sarcoma rarely involves the gastrointestinal tract
    D   weight loss usually signifies a malabsorption state
    E   oesophageal candidiasis responds well to oral nystatin

19   In patients with symptomatic gastro-oesophageal reflux
    A   symptoms are often relieved by eating
    B   normal endoscopy and barium swallow/meal excludes the diagnosis
    C   omeprazole is useful in resistant cases
    D   oesophageal manometry is of diagnostic value
    E   symptoms are precipitated by exercise

20   Toxic dilatation of the colon
    A   is a recognized complication of pseudo-membranous colitis
    B   due to ulcerative colitis, usually responds promptly to intravenous corticosteroids
    C   slowly improves with anti-diarrhoeal agents
    D   is a recognized feature of Hirschsprung's disease
    E   requires barium enema for definitive diagnosis

21   Polycythaemia rubra vera is associated with
    A   an increased incidence of acute myeloid leukaemia
    B   a low leucocyte alkaline phosphatase score
    C   increased secretion of erythropoietin
    D   iron deficiency
    E   an increased incidence of bleeding problems

22   Immune-mediated haemolytic anaemia is
    A   a recognized feature of non-Hodgkin's lymphoma
    B   a recognized complication of penicillin therapy
    C   best treated by blood transfusion
    D   usually associated with a positive direct Coombs' test
    E   a cause of neonatal jaundice

23   Thrombosis is a recognized complication of
    A   antithrombin III deficiency
    B   paroxysmal nocturnal haemoglobinuria
    C   systemic lupus erythematosus
    D   Christmas disease
    E   primary thrombocythaemia

18 A **False**
    B **True**
    C **False**
    D **False**
    E **False**

19 A **False**
    B **False**
    C **True**
    D **False**
    E **True**

20 A **True**
    B **False**
    C **False**
    D **False**
    E **False**

21 A **True**
    B **False**
    C **True**
    D **True**
    E **True**

22 A **True**
    B **True**
    C **False**
    D **True**
    E **True**

23 A **True**
    B **True**
    C **True**
    D **False**
    E **True**

24   In acute myeloid leukaemia
  A   antibiotics should be reserved until infection has been confirmed
  B   relapse is unlikely providing complete remission has occurred
  C   vincristine and prednisolone are the chemotherapeutic drugs of choice
  D   maintenance treatment is of no proven value
  E   preceding myelodysplastic syndrome is a recognized feature

25   In the treatment of post-primary pulmonary tuberculosis
  A   treatment should be withheld until acid- and alcohol-fast bacilli are identified
  B   tuberculin-positive child contacts should receive chemoprophylaxis with isoniazid
  C   hospital admission is necessary for chronic alcoholics
  D   corticosteroids are indicated in hypersensitivity reactions
  E   rifampicin enhances the hypoglycaemic effect of chlorpropamide

26   Characteristic findings in cryptogenic fibrosing alveolitis include
  A   bilateral upper zone crackles
  B   finger and toe clubbing
  C   peak incidence in the 70–80 year age group
  D   pink sputum production
  E   reduced carbon monoxide transfer factor in the early stages

27   In patients with bronchial asthma
  A   the functional residual capacity is reduced in an acute attack
  B   the FEV_1/FVC is often normal between attacks
  C   inhaled corticosteroids have major systemic effects
  D   isolation of *Aspergillus fumigatus* in sputum is an indication for treatment with high-dose steroid therapy
  E   sodium cromoglycate therapy is more effective in children than in adults

28   Recognized pulmonary complications of rheumatoid disease include
  A   reversible airways obstruction
  B   pleural effusion containing cholesterol crystals
  C   primary pulmonary hypertension
  D   lower zone without upper zone fibrosis
  E   nodular shadowing on chest X-ray

24　A　**False**
　　B　**False**
　　C　**False**
　　D　**True**
　　E　**True**

25　A　**False**
　　B　**False**
　　C　**True**
　　D　**True**
　　E　**False**

26　A　**False**
　　B　**True**
　　C　**False**
　　D　**False**
　　E　**True**

27　A　**False**
　　B　**True**
　　C　**False**
　　D　**False**
　　E　**True**

28　A　**False**
　　B　**True**
　　C　**False**
　　D　**False**
　　E　**True**

29   In patients with anterior myocardial infarction
   A   the development of bifascicular block indicates a poor prognosis
   B   intravenous streptokinase given within 6 hours of symptoms onset reduces mortality
   C   the development of complete heart block is an indication for pacemaker insertion
   D   the prophylactic use of subcutaneous heparin is contraindicated
   E   ventricular fibrillation in the first 3 hours, if successfully treated, indicates a poor prognosis

30   On clinical examination
   A   the first heart sound is typically increased in aortic stenosis
   B   the second heart sound is usually diminished in severe mitral stenosis
   C   a blood pressure of 180/100 mmHg in a 70-year-old man excludes significant aortic stenosis
   D   the intensity of the diastolic murmur is a reliable guide to severity in aortic incompetence
   E   the murmur of tricuspid stenosis becomes louder during deep inspiration

31   Features of chronic constrictive pericarditis include
   A   a rise in systolic blood pressure on inspiration
   B   a fall in venous pressure on inspiration
   C   pulsus alternans
   D   ascites
   E   a low pulse pressure

32   Characteristic features of infective endocarditis in the heroin addict include
   A   immune complex nephritis
   B   dental caries
   C   rigors
   D   splenomegaly
   E   lung abscesses

33   The following features usefully help to distinguish hypopituitarism from chronic malnutrition
   A   cold intolerance
   B   amenorrhoea
   C   increased body hair
   D   decreased libido
   E   loss of body fat

29 A **True**
    B **True**
    C **True**
    D **False**
    E **False**

30 A **False**
    B **False**
    C **False**
    D **False**
    E **True**

31 A **False**
    B **False**
    C **False**
    D **True**
    E **True**

32 A **True**
    B **False**
    C **True**
    D **True**
    E **True**

33 A **False**
    B **False**
    C **False**
    D **False**
    E **False**

34 Characteristic features of Graves' thyrotoxicosis include
  A pretibial myxoedema
  B prompt remission with propranolol therapy
  C a lowered serum free tri-iodothyronine in the early stage
  D bilateral exophthalmos
  E a low 4-hour uptake of ^{131}I

35 Galactorrhoea is a recognized feature of
  A spironolactone therapy
  B herpes zoster of the thoracic wall
  C renal carcinoma
  D untreated hypothyroidism
  E ranitidine therapy

36 In diabetic ketoacidosis
  A pneumomediastinum is a recognized complication
  B hydroxybutyrate gives a positive urinary ketostix reaction
  C plasma glucose need not be greater than 18 mmol/l
  D plasma lactate is significantly elevated
  E vomiting should be treated by oral cyclizine

37 In the anaemia associated with rheumatoid arthritis
  A a normochromic normocytic blood film is common
  B hypochromia and microcytosis often does not respond to oral iron
  C an elevated serum ferritin excludes iron deficiency
  D an associated eosinophilia is typical of vasculitis
  E minor splenomegaly can resolve with iron administration

38 Cardiac involvement in rheumatoid arthritis
  A is rare in the absence of a previous history of rheumatic fever
  B is usually apparent as pericarditis
  C is confined to the pericardium and endocardium
  D is seldom evident clinically but common at autopsy
  E results in constrictive pericarditis in some patients

39 D-penicillamine therapy in rheumatoid arthritis
  A usually results in significant improvement in the majority of patients
  B should be discontinued if there is no improvement in 1 year
  C usually produces some clinical improvement within 2 weeks of onset
  D should be stopped if platelet count falls below 50×10^9/l
  E is associated with immune complex nephritis which results in proteinuria

34 A **True**
    B **False**
    C **False**
    D **True**
    E **False**

35 A **False**
    B **True**
    C **True**
    D **True**
    E **False**

36 A **True**
    B **False**
    C **True**
    D **True**
    E **False**

37 A **True**
    B **True**
    C **False**
    D **True**
    E **True**

38 A **False**
    B **True**
    C **False**
    D **True**
    E **True**

39 A **True**
    B **True**
    C **False**
    D **True**
    E **True**

40   Anti-Ro antinuclear antibodies are of diagnostic value in
A   chronic active hepatitis
B   systemic sclerosis
C   CREST syndrome
D   mixed connective tissue disease
E   primary Sjögren's disease (sicca syndrome)

41   The following are typical features of motor neurone disease
A   dysarthria
B   muscle fasciculation
C   early sphincter involvement
D   loss of taste
E   diplopia

42   Common presenting features of multiple sclerosis include
A   diplopia
B   dysphasia
C   painful uniocular visual impairment
D   numbness of the lower limbs
E   homonymous hemianopia

43   Unilateral facial nerve paralysis is a recognized feature of
A   herpes zoster infection
B   motor neurone disease
C   migrainous neuralgia
D   acoustic neuroma
E   cholesteatoma

44   Features favouring a lesion in the brain stem rather than in the cerebral cortex include the presence of
A   grasp reflex
B   dysphasia
C   vertigo
D   dysphagia
E   nystagmus

45   In Chagas' disease
A   *Trypanosoma cruzi* is the causative agent
B   the typical route of infection is the conjunctiva and mucous membranes
C   megaoesophagus and megacolon are the result of destruction of Meissner's submucous plexus
D   the monkey is a recognized animal reservoir
E   myocarditis takes more than 2 years to develop

40 A **False**
   B **False**
   C **False**
   D **True**
   E **True**

41 A **True**
   B **True**
   C **False**
   D **False**
   E **False**

42 A **True**
   B **False**
   C **True**
   D **True**
   E **False**

43 A **True**
   B **True**
   C **False**
   D **True**
   E **True**

44 A **False**
   B **False**
   C **True**
   D **True**
   E **True**

45 A **True**
   B **True**
   C **False**
   D **False**
   E **False**

46   Typical features of poliomyelitis include
  A   DNA virus infection
  B   muscle pain in the limbs and back
  C   an increase in polymorphs in CSF soon after onset
  D   sensory signs which progress rapidly
  E   bladder dysfunction which recovers rapidly

47   In the acquired immune deficiency syndrome (AIDS) as experienced in Europe and North America
  A   most sufferers are intravenous drug abusers
  B   infectivity is greater than that of hepatitis B
  C   the majority of babies born to infected mothers become infected
  D   the cell most impaired is the B lymphocyte
  E   toxoplasmosis pneumonia is a recognized complication

48   The following statements about malaria are correct
  A   the pattern of fever associated with *P. malariae* infection is a useful diagnostic aid
  B   *P. falciparum* in South-East Asia is normally chloroquine-sensitive
  C   *P. falciparum* infection can relapse after effective treatment because of persistent liver forms
  D   rupture of the spleen is commonest in *P. vivax* infections
  E   the usual cause of death in *P. falciparum* is severe haemolytic anaemia

49   Nail dystrophy is typically associated with
  A   epidermolysis bullosa
  B   lichen planus
  C   alopecia areata
  D   erythema nodosum
  E   psoriasis

50   Physiological functions of the kidney include the production of
  A   aldosterone
  B   erythropoietin
  C   atrial natriuretic peptide
  D   25-hydroxycholecalciferol
  E   prostaglandin E2

51   Exposure to
  A   toluene di-isocyanate produces asthma in susceptible subjects
  B   asbestos predisposes to pulmonary tuberculosis
  C   mercury poisoning typically causes ataxia
  D   carbon monoxide poisoning causes parkinsonism
  E   nickel causes dermatitis only in areas in direct contact with the metal

46 A **False**
    B **True**
    C **True**
    D **False**
    E **True**

47 A **False**
    B **False**
    C **False**
    D **False**
    E **True**

48 A **False**
    B **False**
    C **False**
    D **True**
    E **False**

49 A **True**
    B **True**
    C **True**
    D **False**
    E **True**

50 A **False**
    B **True**
    C **False**
    D **False**
    E **True**

51 A **True**
    B **False**
    C **True**
    D **True**
    E **False**

52   **Somatic symptoms of depressive illness typically include**
    A   insomnia
    B   headache
    C   diarrhoea
    D   nocturia
    E   amenorrhoea

53   **Typical features of rapid eye movement sleep include**
    A   slow regular respiration
    B   paradoxical depression of muscle tone
    C   increased heart rate and blood pressure
    D   penile erection and perspiration
    E   progressive slowing of the EEG

54   **The following statements about drug treatment in Parkinson's disease are correct**
    A   levodopa should be used in combination with carbidopa
    B   amantadine should be withdrawn if unhelpful within 1 week
    C   benztropine is useful in controlling the tremor
    D   drug therapy is better given and more effective at the onset of mild symptoms
    E   bromocriptine is particularly effective in drug-induced parkinsonism

55   **Typical causes of urinary incontinence include**
    A   diuretic therapy
    B   severe Parkinson's disease
    C   benign prostatic hyperplasia
    D   normal pressure hydrocephalus
    E   faecal impaction

56   **The typical features of senile dementia include**
    A   dyspraxia
    B   alteration in emotional and behavioural characteristics
    C   paranoid delusions
    D   auditory hallucinations
    E   endogenous depression

57   **In the brain stem control of breathing**
    A   fever reduces the sensitivity of the respiratory centre
    B   only central chemoreceptors are sensitive to arterial PCO_2
    C   peripheral chemoreceptors are sensitive only to arterial PO_2
    D   chronic alveolar hypoventilation decreases sensitivity to arterial PO_2
    E   limb, chest wall and pulmonary stretch receptors stimulate ventilation during exercise

52 A **True**
    B **True**
    C **False**
    D **False**
    E **False**

53 A **False**
    B **True**
    C **True**
    D **True**
    E **False**

54 A **True**
    B **True**
    C **True**
    D **False**
    E **False**

55 A **True**
    B **True**
    C **True**
    D **True**
    E **True**

56 A **False**
    B **True**
    C **True**
    D **False**
    E **False**

57 A **False**
    B **False**
    C **True**
    D **True**
    E **True**

58 During a standard Valsalva manoeuvre
   A   an increase in the pulse rate suggests left ventricular failure
   B   forced inspiration is undertaken against a closed glottis
   C   on release, the blood pressure falls and a reflex bradycardia occurs
   D   an increase in heart rate with a reduction in pulse pressure is a normal finding
   E   the blood pressure and pulse rate normally rise soon after straining is terminated

59 Bilirubin is
   A   derived exclusively from the breakdown of haemoglobin
   B   transported in plasma bound to the beta-globulins
   C   conjugated in the endoplasmic reticulum of the hepatocyte
   D   rendered water-soluble by the process of glucuronidation
   E   normally excreted as stercobilinogen in faeces and urobilinogen in the urine

60 In delayed hypersensitivity reactions
   A   T cells recruit macrophages in the development of the response
   B   provoking infectious agents are typically extracellular
   C   antigen within the macrophage persists undestroyed
   D   such as contact eczema, sensitizing agents behave as haptens
   E   Langerhan's cells in the dermis present the antigen in eczema

58 A **False**
   B **False**
   C **False**
   D **True**
   E **False**

59 A **False**
   B **False**
   C **True**
   D **True**
   E **True**

60 A **True**
   B **False**
   C **True**
   D **True**
   E **True**